Dr. Barbara Bible:

Exploring DNA, Nutrition, Detoxification, Herbal Remedies, Diabetes Management, and Water Therapy with O'Neill's Teachings

Simon Jr. Jackson

Contents

Acknowledgment and Disclaimer

This book, while inspired by the teachings and philosophy of Barbara O'Neill, is an original work and has been written and published in full compliance with copyright laws. It is important to note that while I have drawn inspiration from Barbara O'Neill's holistic approach to health and well-being, the content within these pages is the result of my own research, experiences, and interpretations.

The ideas, strategies, and recommendations presented in this book are not endorsed by, nor do they represent the views or teachings of Barbara O'Neill directly. This work is intended to pay homage to the insights she has provided into natural health and wholesome living while offering my unique perspective and understanding on these topics.

The aim of this book is to provide valuable information and insights to those seeking guidance on a journey to better health and well-being, using the inspiration provided by Barbara O'Neill as a starting point. It should be read and utilized as a separate entity, distinct from Barbara O'Neill's own publications and materials.

This book is not affiliated with, authorized, sponsored, or otherwise endorsed by Barbara O'Neill. All content herein is provided for informational purposes only and should not be construed as medical advice. Readers are encouraged to consult healthcare professionals for advice on their individual health needs.

Introduction

As you hold "Dr. Barbara Bible" in your hands, you are not just holding a book; you are holding a gateway to a journey of transformation and discovery. My name is Simon Jr. Jackson, and it has been my honor and privilege to bring to you this compendium of knowledge and wisdom, a tribute to the unparalleled insights of Dr. Barbara O'Neill in the dimension of natural health and wholesome living.

This book is the culmination of a profound exploration, not just for me as a writer, but for all of us who seek deeper understanding and harmony with our bodies and nature. In these pages, I have endeavored to encapsulate the essence of Dr. O'Neill's teachings, her philosophy of life, and her unwavering commitment to holistic health. It is a travel that delves into the mysteries of nutrition, the art of detoxification, the power of herbal remedies, and the foundational pillars of a healthy lifestyle.

My hope is that as you cross through each chapter, you will find not just information, but inspiration. This book is an invitation to embark on your own path of discovery, to explore new ways of living, eating, and thinking. It is an encouragement to embrace a lifestyle that is in harmony with nature and to discover the joy and vitality that comes with it.

I invite you to approach this book with an open mind and heart. Let the pages speak to you, challenge you, and guide you. May this book enrich your life, bring you closer to the essence of true health, and inspire you to embrace the beauty of a life lived in harmony with nature.

Thank you for joining me on these remarkable studies. May the insights you gain here light your path to health, happiness, and holistic well-being.

Who is Dr. Barbara?

Barbara O'Neill, born on July 28, 1953, in Australia, has had a significant career as a naturopath and nutritionist, known for her work as the Health Director of Misty Mountain Health Retreat. Her studies into natural health began from an early age, growing up in a family that valued the healing power of nature. This upbringing instilled in her a deep-rooted passion for natural remedies and alternative therapies, shaping her life's work and dedication to the field of holistic wellness.

Her educational background includes obtaining degrees in health science and naturopathy, which enabled her to become a certified naturopath and nutritionist. Her commitment to continuous learning and research is evident in her extensive knowledge of natural healing and nutrition.

Throughout her career, Barbara has made significant contributions to the field of holistic wellness through her establishment of wellness retreats and educational seminars. These initiatives offer individuals unique opportunities to immerse themselves in the healing power of nature, proper nutrition, and healthy lifestyle practices. Her retreats and seminars are known for being transformative experiences that leave participants rejuvenated and equipped with practical knowledge for leading healthier lives.

Barbara's advocacy for natural healing methods has also gained her a dedicated following on social media platforms, where she shares health tips, insights, and inspirational stories. Her active presence on these platforms has allowed her to connect with a global community of wellness enthusiasts, making her a trusted source of health information and inspiration.

As an author, Barbara has written several books and publications on various topics related to holistic health, including nutrition and detoxification. Her literary works have inspired many readers and are promoted and discussed extensively through her social media channels.

Barbara's biography is a testament to the transformative power of dedication and passion for natural healing. Her unwavering commitment to helping others live healthier, happier lives has left an enduring legacy in the field of holistic wellness, extending beyond physical spaces into the digital universe, where her social media influence continues to grow.

Her path wasn't just shaped by academic study but also enriched by hands-on experiences and a heartfelt connection to the healing arts.

As an educator, Barbara has always stood out for her ability to demystify the complexities of health and nutrition, making them accessible and understandable to people from all walks of life. Her approach is characterized by a blend of scientific rigor and a deep respect for traditional wisdom, a combination that has endeared her to both the academic community and the general public.

Barbara's philosophy on health and wellness is holistic and integrative, recognizing the interconnectedness of all aspects of health – physical, mental, emotional, and environmental. She advocates for a lifestyle that is in harmony with nature, emphasizing the importance of a balanced diet, the healing power of herbs, the benefits of detoxification, and the crucial role of lifestyle factors like exercise and sleep.

With a relentless thirst for knowledge, Barbara augmented her formal education with a wealth of self-study and research, delving into ancient healing traditions and modern scientific findings alike.

One of the cornerstones of her career has been her emphasis on preventative health. Barbara has consistently advocated for the proactive maintenance of health through natural means - a balanced diet, the use of medicinal herbs, regular physical activity, and stress management. Her approach goes beyond treating symptoms, focusing instead on nurturing the body's inherent ability to heal and maintain balance.

In her clinical practice, she has worked closely with individuals, helping them to navigate their health challenges through natural therapies. Her expertise in herbal remedies and nutritional counseling has been a beacon of hope for many seeking alternative or complementary approaches to conventional medical treatments.

Chapter 1: DNA and Disease Prevention

The revelation of DNA and its profound significance as the genetic code residing within the confines of every single cell has initiated a paradigm shift in our understanding of life itself. This groundbreaking revelation, while aligning with some aspects of Darwin's evolutionary theory, also serves to challenge certain facets of his paradigm. DNA, often referred to as the molecule of life, unravels the intricate secrets of existence, shedding light on the complex mechanisms that underpin the development, functioning, and even the potential deterioration of living organisms.

At the heart of this revolution in biology is the profound insight that DNA encodes the instructions for the formation and functioning of all living beings. It is the architectural blueprint that orchestrates the symphony of life, guiding the intricate dance of cellular processes. This newfound understanding has led us to acknowledge that life is not merely the result of random genetic mutations, as proposed by Darwinian evolution, but rather a meticulously scripted genetic masterpiece.

However, while the discovery of DNA has unveiled many of the mysteries of existence, it has also brought to the forefront a paradox that challenges conventional scientific thought. It is the paradox of epigenetics—a field of study that has ushered in a new era of biological exploration. Epigenetics reveals that our lifestyles, choices, and environments wield significant influence over our genetic destiny. In essence, it suggests that genetics may load the gun, but it is our lifestyle that ultimately pulls the trigger.

This revelation has profound implications for our understanding of health, disease, and the aging process. It compels us to recognize that our genes are not immutable dictates but rather dynamic entities that respond to the way we live our lives. Epigenetics elucidates the intricate interplay between nature and nurture, highlighting the remarkable adaptability of our genetic makeup in response to external stimuli.

Consider, for a moment, the concept of premature aging and disease. It is a notion that has plagued humanity for centuries, as we witness the relentless march of time and its seemingly inevitable toll on our bodies. However, the insights garnered from the study of epigenetics invite us to question this inevitability. The human body, it appears, was not designed to succumb to the ravages of time as swiftly as it often does.

The very essence of our biological makeup suggests that our bodies possess an innate resilience—a remarkable ability to heal, rejuvenate, and withstand the challenges of aging. Nature has endowed us with a biological arsenal that, under ideal circumstances, equips us to maintain vitality and ward off the encroachment of diseases. It is a testament to the intricate design of the human body—a design that seemingly defies the relentless march of time.

Yet, herein lies the conundrum. If our bodies possess such remarkable restorative capabilities, why do we witness the premature aging of individuals and the proliferation of diseases that often accompany the passage of time? Could there be external factors at play—factors that conspire against the innate wisdom of our biology?

The revelations of epigenetics point us toward a resounding affirmative. They beckon us to explore the external influences that impede the natural course of health and vitality. It becomes apparent that the detriments to our well-being are not solely the result of genetic preordainment but rather the consequence of our choices, our environments, and our lifestyles.

In this narrative, the human body emerges as a resilient fortress, besieged by the onslaught of modern living. It beseeches us to consider the impact of our dietary choices, the quality of our sleep, the levels of stress we endure, and the toxins we encounter daily. These elements, it appears, have the potential to accelerate the aging process and open the door to the onset of diseases.

It is a stark reminder that the secrets of health and longevity are not confined to the confines of our genes but are intrinsically linked to the choices we make on a daily basis. We hold the power to influence our genetic destiny, to navigate the intricate labyrinth of epigenetic pathways, and to chart a course toward vibrant health and well-being.

The discovery of DNA as the genetic code within every cell has ushered in an era of profound scientific understanding. It has challenged Darwin's theory of evolution while revealing the intricate secrets of life. Epigenetics, a burgeoning field of study, has unveiled the profound impact of lifestyle choices on our genes, reinforcing the idea that genetics provides the blueprint, but it is our way of life that determines the outcome.

Moreover, the revelation that the human body possesses innate healing abilities, and that premature aging and disease may be influenced by external factors, underscores the importance of our choices and environments in shaping our health. It is a call to action—a call to embrace the wisdom of our biology and harness the power of epigenetics to lead lives filled with vitality and well-being.

Nutritional Factors and Disease

In the intricate tapestry of human health, there exists a profound connection between our nutritional choices and the state of our well-being. This connection transcends the mere act of eating; it delves deep into the very essence of our existence, where the building blocks of life are woven together. It is within this domain that we encounter the pivotal role of nutritional factors in determining the course of our health and the onset of disease.

At the heart of this revelation lies a staggering statistic—92% of DNA damage is caused by a mineral deficiency. This single statistic serves as a clarion call to awaken us to the paramount importance of proper nutrition for our overall health. It is a statistic that unveils a profound truth: our bodies are intricately intertwined with the nutrients they receive. These nutrients are not mere fuel for our physical machinery; they are the very architects of our cellular existence.

Consider for a moment the analogy of constructing a building. Just as a skilled builder requires the right materials to erect a sturdy and resilient structure, our bodies require proper nutrition to heal, repair, and flourish. Every cell, tissue, and organ within us relies on a delicate balance of minerals, vitamins, and nutrients to function optimally. Without this balance, our bodies become susceptible to the ravages of disease, as the very fabric of our DNA becomes compromised.

The decline in the mineral content of Australian soil over the past 50 years, as documented by Dr. Robert Thompson in his book "The Calcium Lie," paints a stark picture of the challenges we face. The mineral content has decreased by a staggering 50%, resulting in nutrient deficiencies not only in the plants that draw sustenance from this soil but also in the humans who consume these plants. This decline in mineral richness sets the stage for a cascade of health issues, as our bodies struggle to obtain the essential elements they require.

Nourishment, in its truest sense, is not merely a matter of filling our stomachs; it is an act of providing our bodies with the raw materials they need to thrive. Imagine constructing a magnificent structure without the requisite bricks, mortar, and steel. Similarly, our bodies cannot embark on the journey of self-healing and vitality without the foundational elements of proper nutrition.

Yet, the story of nutrition's impact on health extends beyond the realm of deficiency; it delves into the intricate relationship between our dietary choices and the presence of disease. It beckons us to explore the shadows where mold, that insidious intruder, lurks. It is a connection that medicine, in its conventional wisdom, often overlooks or chooses to ignore.

Mold, that silent companion of dampness and decay, has been linked to a myriad of health issues. Its insidious presence can trigger allergies, respiratory problems, and a host of mysterious ailments. Yet, within the annals of modern medicine, mold remains an unspoken adversary—a specter that haunts the lives of many without receiving the acknowledgment it deserves.

Why, you might ask, does medicine turn a blind eye to mold's insinuations? The answer lies in the uncomfortable truth that acknowledging mold's role would also require us to confront the darker side of pharmaceutical interventions. Mold thrives in environments influenced by antibiotics, statin drugs, contraceptive pills, and cortisone—medications that are meant to heal but inadvertently contribute to the mold's presence within us.

In the pursuit of symptom alleviation, we unwittingly create fertile ground for mold's proliferation. This intricate dance between medication and mold is a silent narrative that often eludes our awareness. It is a reminder that the complexities of health and disease extend far beyond the confines of a single pill or prescription. It is a testament to the interconnectedness of our choices, our environment, and our well-being.

Nutrition offers more than mere nourishment; it presents a critical path to healing and guarding against illness. In this sphere, the lack of vital minerals poses a threat to our genetic integrity, and the diminishing mineral content in our soils echoes through what we eat. Moreover, the subtle yet significant impact of mold, often overshadowed by the prominence of pharmaceutical solutions, influences our health. Our exploration in this field involves choices about our diet, the essential nutrients we focus on, and the treatments we opt for. This exploration is an invitation to rethink our approach to nutrition and acknowledge its essential role in our pursuit of wellness and vigor. It's a journey that highlights a fundamental truth: feeding ourselves goes beyond simple consumption—it's a meaningful act of self-care with the potential to transform our lives and open the door to a healthier, more vibrant existence.

Microbial Composition and Health

Within the intricate ecosystem of our body lies considerable complexity, in fact Barbara argues that the body is a space in which the very essence of our health and vitality is intricately intertwined. It begins in the depths of our gastrointestinal tract, where the cells lining this intricate passageway undergo a constant process of rebirth and renewal. This phenomenon, often unnoticed in the hustle and bustle of our daily lives, carries profound implications for our well-being.

Imagine, for a moment, the cells that line your gastrointestinal tract as diligent workers in a continuous cycle of construction and renovation. These cells, like tireless builders, are engaged in a relentless effort to maintain the integrity of this vital passageway. They are the guardians of your digestive system, ensuring that it functions optimally to support your health.

The significance of this process cannot be overstated, for it underscores the critical importance of caring for our digestive system. In a world filled with distractions and fast-paced living, we often take our gastrointestinal health for granted. Yet, within this ceaseless renewal lies a reminder—an invitation to nurture and protect this essential component of our well-being.

In the midst of our daily lives, where the hum of electronic devices surrounds us, there exists a subtle but potent force—an electronic field. It is a force that permeates our modern existence, woven into the fabric of our technological age. Yet, beneath its convenience and allure, there lies a shadow—a shadow cast by the growing body of research that unveils the potential dangers of electronic field exposure.

"Be very careful of your electronic field exposure," cautions a voice from the depths of knowledge. It echoes the sentiment of 80,000 research papers that illuminate the risks concealed to electronic devices. These papers, borne from the collective wisdom of scientific inquiry, stand as sentinels, guarding the gates to our well-being.

Delve deeper into the mysteries of our bodies, and you will discover a revelation—a revelation that challenges our perception of ourselves. Within the human body, there exist not merely cells but an entire microcosm—an intricate tapestry of microorganisms that outnumber our cells tenfold. These microorganisms, so numerous and diverse, have found their stronghold in the very core of our being—the gastrointestinal tract.

In contemplating this astonishing fact, we are beckoned to consider a profound notion: that in terms of our microbial composition, we may be more akin to plants than animals. It is a concept that transcends the boundaries of traditional classification, inviting us to embrace the interconnectedness of all life forms. Within our bodies, a delicate equilibrium exists—a harmony between our cells and the myriad microorganisms that share our existence.

As we journey through the annals of medical history, the wisdom of ancient healers resounds—a wisdom encapsulated in the words of Hippocrates. "All disease begins in the gut," declared this sage of antiquity, casting a timeless light on the importance of our gastrointestinal health. These words, uttered centuries ago, remain as relevant today as they were in the days of antiquity.

Hippocrates' proclamation serves as a beacon, illuminating the path to wellness. It underscores the significance of maintaining a healthy gut microbiome—a diverse and thriving community of microorganisms that call our gastrointestinal tract home. It is within this microbial system that the seeds of health and disease are sown—something that demands our care, attention, and respect.

In the intricate dance of our bodily functions, the gastrointestinal tract takes center stage—a stage upon which the cells that line its walls perform a symphony of renewal and protection. It is a stage upon which the electronic fields of our modern world cast their shadows, urging us to tread carefully. It is a stage where the microbial inhabitants outnumber our own cells, prompting us to reevaluate our place in the grand tapestry of life. And it is a stage where the wisdom of ancient healers resonates, reminding us that true health begins in the gut.

As we navigate the labyrinth of our bodies, let us heed these revelations, for they offer profound insights into the art of living well. Let us honor the ceaseless renewal of our gastrointestinal cells, for they are the sentinels of our digestive health. Let us approach the electronic fields of our age with mindfulness, for their effects on our well-being are not to be taken lightly. Let us embrace our microbial companions, recognizing the interconnectedness of all life. And above all, let us cherish the wisdom of Hippocrates, for it is a timeless guide on our journey toward health and vitality.

Within the depths of our digestive system lies a world teeming with life—a bustling community of microorganisms that have long been misunderstood and underestimated. For years, these tiny inhabitants of our gut have been cast as villains in the drama of human health, accused of causing havoc and digestive distress. Yet, recent revelations have shattered this perception, revealing a truth that challenges the very essence of our relationship with these microorganisms—they are not the enemy, but rather indispensable allies in our quest for well-being.

The human gut is a complex and dynamic ecosystem, home to an astonishing diversity of microorganisms. These microscopic residents include bacteria, viruses, fungi, and other microbial entities, collectively referred to as the gut microbiota. While their existence has been acknowledged for centuries, it is only in recent years that we have begun to uncover the profound impact they wield over our health.

One of the most astonishing aspects of the gut microbiota is its sheer abundance. The numbers are staggering—there are ten times more microorganisms residing within our gastrointestinal tract than there are human cells in our entire body. This revelation alone challenges our perception of self, suggesting that we may be more plant-like than animal-like in terms of our microbial composition.

The importance of these microorganisms cannot be overstated, as they play a pivotal role in the breakdown, absorption, and protection of the food we consume. They are the silent workers behind the scenes, diligently breaking down complex carbohydrates, proteins, and other nutrients into forms that our bodies can absorb and utilize. Without their tireless efforts, the process of digestion and nutrient absorption would be a far more arduous and inefficient endeavor.

Yet, the significance of our gut microbiota extends beyond their digestive duties. They serve as guardians of our well-being, standing sentinel against harmful substances that may find their way into our digestive tract. These microorganisms, in their collective wisdom, protect us from potentially pathogenic invaders, helping to maintain a delicate balance within our gut.

This newfound understanding of the gut microbiota challenges the age-old notion that all microorganisms are to be feared and eradicated. Instead, it compels us to reevaluate our relationship with these tiny inhabitants, recognizing that they are not adversaries but partners in our journey toward health.

In the words of the ancient Greek physician Hippocrates, "Let food be your medicine and medicine be your food." This sage advice takes on a deeper resonance in light of our evolving understanding of the gut microbiota. It underscores the pivotal role of nutrition in not only fueling our bodies but also nurturing the trillions of microorganisms that reside within us.

The health of our gut is paramount, for it directly influences our overall well-being. An imbalanced or disturbed gut microbiota can lead to a cascade of health issues, including digestive disorders, immune system dysfunction, and even mental health concerns. It is a stark reminder that the intricate dance between our diet and our gut health is a fundamental aspect of our vitality.

As we navigate the intricacies of our digestive system and the crucial role played by the gut microbiota, we are compelled to view these microorganisms through a new lens—one that recognizes their essential contributions to our health. It is a paradigm shift that challenges long-held beliefs and invites us to embrace the notion that within our own bodies, a thriving microbial metropolis exists—one that, when nurtured and respected, can be a powerful ally in our pursuit of well-being.

In conclusion, the microorganisms that inhabit our gut are not adversaries to be feared but allies to be cherished. They play a vital role in the breakdown and absorption of our food, as well as in the protection of our digestive tract. The health of our gut is intricately linked to our overall well-being, underscoring the wisdom of Hippocrates' advice to let food be our medicine. As we continue to unravel the mysteries of the gut microbiota, we are poised to unlock new avenues for enhancing our health and vitality, all within our own bodies.

Habits

Within the intricate tapestry of life, the fundamental blueprint that dictates our existence lies in the mysterious DNA. This double-helix structure, comprised of nucleotide bases and coiled into a spiraling ladder, carries the genetic code that orchestrates the symphony of our existence. Yet, beyond the conventional understanding of genetics, lies a captivating revelation—one that transcends the boundaries of traditional science and delves into the profound interplay between our lifestyle choices and the very essence of our being.

In the realm of genetics, the prevailing belief was once that our DNA was an immutable script, an unalterable manuscript passed down through generations—an unchangeable legacy that determined our health and predispositions. However, the emerging field of epigenetics has shattered this paradigm, illuminating a path where our habits and choices hold the power to inscribe their mark upon the delicate pages of our genetic code.

Epigenetics, a term derived from the Greek words "epi" (above) and "genetics," explores the intricate molecular mechanisms that reside above our genes, orchestrating their activity like a conductor guiding an orchestra. It unveils the profound truth that our lifestyle choices, environmental exposures, and even emotional experiences can exert a significant influence on the way our genes are expressed. In essence, epigenetics reveals that while genetics may load the gun, it is our lifestyle that ultimately pulls the trigger.

Imagine our DNA as a grand library, with each gene representing a unique book. In the conventional genetic paradigm, these books were considered static and unchangeable. However, epigenetics introduces the concept of "gene expression," which is akin to opening and reading these books. Gene expression determines whether a particular gene is active or silenced, thereby influencing the traits or conditions it governs.

This intricate process of gene expression is regulated by a group of chemical modifications known as epigenetic marks. These marks can attach themselves to the DNA molecule or the proteins that package it, altering the accessibility of genes. They act as molecular switches, deciding which genes are turned on and which remain dormant. In this way, epigenetics introduces a layer of complexity and adaptability to our genetic code that was once thought impossible.

Now, consider the choices we make in our daily lives—our dietary preferences, physical activity levels, exposure to environmental toxins, and even our emotional well-being. These choices, it turns out, have the remarkable capacity to influence the placement and removal of these epigenetic marks. They can dictate whether a gene linked to disease remains dormant or becomes active, thereby influencing our susceptibility to health conditions.

The foods we consume contain a myriad of bioactive compounds, some of which can affect our epigenetic marks. Certain nutrients, such as folate, vitamin B12, and methyl donors found in foods like broccoli and spinach, play a crucial role in the addition of methyl groups to our DNA—a process known as DNA methylation. This epigenetic modification can silence genes associated with inflammation and disease, thereby promoting better health.

Conversely, a diet high in processed foods, saturated fats, and sugar can lead to epigenetic changes that activate genes linked to chronic diseases like diabetes, obesity, and cardiovascular conditions. This illustrates the profound impact of dietary choices on our epigenetic landscape and, subsequently, our health.

But epigenetic influence extends beyond our dietary habits. The stress we experience, for instance, can leave a lasting imprint on our genetic code. Chronic stress triggers the release of stress hormones, which can lead to epigenetic modifications that impact mental health and even future generations. This phenomenon highlights the interconnectedness of our experiences and their enduring effects on our genetic legacy.

Moreover, environmental exposures, such as pollutants, chemicals, and radiation, can also introduce epigenetic changes that influence health outcomes. These factors emphasize the importance of creating environments that safeguard our genetic well-being and that of generations to come.

In the context of our future generations, epigenetics unveils a captivating narrative. It suggests that the choices we make today can echo through the corridors of time, influencing the health and well-being of our descendants. Epigenetic marks, imprinted by our lifestyle choices, can be inherited by our offspring, potentially impacting their susceptibility to diseases or conditions we may never personally experience.

Consider the profound implications of this revelation for expecting parents. A mother's diet, stress levels, and exposures during pregnancy can shape the epigenetic landscape of her unborn child, influencing their health and development. It underscores the responsibility of individuals to make choices that foster a healthy genetic legacy for their progeny.

In essence, epigenetics invites us to recognize the remarkable agency we possess in shaping our genetic destiny. It empowers us with the knowledge that our habits and choices can potentially rewrite the narrative encoded in our DNA. It prompts us to embark on a journey of mindful living—a path where our actions today reverberate through the annals of our genetic history.

As we traverse this landscape of epigenetics, we are called to embrace the profound interconnectedness of our choices, our genes, and the legacy we leave for future generations. It is a narrative that transcends the boundaries of traditional genetics and beckons us to embark on a voyage of self-discovery and empowerment—a voyage where our choices hold the power to sculpt the destiny of our DNA and the health of generations yet to come.

Caffeine

Caffeine, most of the time is just a habit, often regarded as a harmless and ubiquitous stimulant, conceals a paradoxical truth beneath its innocuous facade. This truth is unveiled when one delves into the harrowing world of withdrawals, where it becomes apparent that caffeine withdrawals can rival, and in some instances surpass, the intensity of withdrawals from notorious substances such as methamphetamines, heroin, methadone, alcohol, and tobacco. It is a revelation that sheds light on the profound impact caffeine can exert on our physiological and psychological well-being.

To appreciate the gravity of this revelation, one must first comprehend the widespread prevalence of caffeine consumption in modern society. Coffee, tea, energy drinks, and even certain medications all contribute to the daily caffeine intake of countless individuals worldwide. It has become an integral part of our daily rituals—a morning elixir that promises alertness and vitality. Yet, beneath its seemingly innocuous allure lies a potent psychoactive substance that our bodies can become profoundly accustomed to.

The process of caffeine addiction begins with regular consumption. As individuals indulge in their daily doses of caffeine, their bodies adjust to the presence of this stimulant. It becomes a routine—a ritualistic act that provides a boost of energy, heightened alertness, and a sense of wakefulness. However, beneath the surface, caffeine is subtly altering the delicate balance of neurotransmitters and hormones in the brain.

Over time, the body adapts to the constant influx of caffeine by increasing the number of adenosine receptors—a pivotal player in regulating sleep and wakefulness. Adenosine is a neurotransmitter that promotes relaxation and sleepiness when it binds to its receptors. Caffeine, being structurally similar to adenosine, competes for these receptors and effectively blocks adenosine's calming effects. The result is increased wakefulness and alertness.

However, this adaptation comes at a cost. As the body accommodates caffeine's presence by upregulating adenosine receptors, it becomes more reliant on caffeine to maintain normal levels of alertness. A vicious cycle ensues, where individuals find themselves increasingly dependent on caffeine to stave off fatigue and drowsiness. This dependence is the first step towards caffeine addiction.

The true revelation emerges when individuals attempt to break free from the clutches of caffeine—a feat that can plunge them into the throes of withdrawal. It is here that the shocking intensity of caffeine withdrawals comes to the fore, eclipsing the challenges posed by withdrawals from substances that are traditionally associated with severe dependency.

Withdrawals from caffeine, often characterized by symptoms such as pounding headaches, extreme fatigue, irritability, and intense cravings, can be excruciatingly debilitating. It is not uncommon for individuals attempting to quit caffeine to experience a profound sense of malaise and discomfort, which can extend for days or even weeks. This is where the paradox of caffeine withdrawals becomes apparent—withdrawals from a substance often perceived as mild can manifest as a harrowing ordeal.

Comparing caffeine withdrawals to withdrawals from substances like methamphetamines, heroin, methadone, alcohol, and tobacco sheds light on the magnitude of this revelation. While the withdrawal experiences associated with these substances are unquestionably arduous and challenging, caffeine withdrawals stand out for their intensity, especially in the short term. The relentless headaches, extreme fatigue, and irritability that accompany caffeine withdrawals can be so debilitating that they rival the severity of withdrawals from highly addictive drugs.

This paradoxical revelation serves as a stark reminder of the pervasive influence of caffeine in our lives and the potential consequences of its overconsumption. It highlights the need for individuals to be mindful of their caffeine intake and to recognize the signs of dependency. Moreover, it underscores the importance of approaching caffeine consumption with moderation and an awareness of its potential withdrawal effects.

The revelation that caffeine withdrawals can be more extreme than withdrawals from methamphetamines, heroin, methadone, alcohol, and tobacco challenges our preconceived notions about caffeine's impact on our well-being. It serves as a cautionary tale, reminding us of the potent influence caffeine can wield over our bodies and minds. This insight urges us to approach caffeine consumption with prudence, recognizing its potential for dependency and the intensity of its withdrawals. It is a revelation that invites us to reevaluate our relationship with this ubiquitous stimulant and prioritize our physical and mental health.

Smoking

Amidst the labyrinthine intricacies of human health, few topics carry the weight of consequence as heavily as the impact of smoking—a habit that extends its pernicious influence far beyond the confines of an individual's lungs. Studying genetics, it unravels a narrative that spans generations, where the choices made by one reverberate through the delicate strands of DNA, affecting not only the smoker but also their progeny.

For decades, the link between smoking and lung cancer has been well-established, casting a long shadow over the health of those who partake in this perilous habit. However, the ramifications of smoking transcend the development of lung cancer, casting an insidious net over the very essence of life—our genetic code.

Within the nucleus of every cell, our DNA resides—a complex tapestry of nucleotide bases, genes, and chromosomes that orchestrate the symphony of our existence. It is the blueprint of life, the repository of genetic information passed down through generations. Yet, the act of smoking, a seemingly innocuous indulgence, has the power to cast a pall over this delicate genetic manuscript.

Pregnancy, a time of profound vulnerability and potential, offers a poignant example of the far-reaching consequences of smoking. When a pregnant woman smokes, the toxic compounds present in cigarette smoke infiltrate her bloodstream, surging through the placenta and into the developing fetus. This ominous journey carries with it a payload of harm, not only to the expectant mother but to the nascent life growing within her.

One of the most unsettling revelations of smoking during pregnancy lies in its ability to inflict lasting damage upon the DNA of the unborn child. Our genetic code, while resilient, is not impervious to the onslaught of harmful substances. Cigarette smoke contains a sinister amalgamation of carcinogens, mutagens, and toxins, some of which have the power to directly affect the DNA of the developing fetus.

At the heart of this genetic transformation lies a process known as DNA methylation—an epigenetic modification that involves the addition of methyl groups to specific regions of DNA. In essence, it acts as a molecular switch, determining whether a gene is active or silenced. DNA methylation plays a pivotal role in gene regulation, and alterations in this process can have profound implications for health.

Smoking during pregnancy has been linked to aberrant DNA methylation patterns in the developing fetus. Specifically, it can lead to the hypermethylation of genes—a phenomenon where methyl groups are added excessively, silencing the expression of these genes. This can disrupt normal developmental processes and predispose the child to a host of health issues.

Among the affected genes are those responsible for lung development, immune function, and neurological processes. As a result, children born to mothers who smoked during pregnancy may face an increased risk of respiratory problems, weakened immune systems, and even neurodevelopmental disorders.

The insidious nature of smoking's genetic impact is further underscored by its potential to affect future generations. While the immediate consequences may manifest in the child born to a smoking mother, the genetic changes wrought by smoking can extend their reach to subsequent generations.

Epigenetic modifications, including DNA methylation patterns, can be heritable, passed down from parent to child. This means that the genetic legacy of smoking can endure, potentially influencing the health of grandchildren and great-grandchildren. It is a haunting testament to the enduring legacy of our choices—a legacy that transcends the boundaries of time and stretches its influence across the vast expanse of genetic history.

The question that arises is not merely one of individual choice but of collective responsibility. It prompts us to ponder the implications of our actions not only for ourselves but for the generations that follow. The pregnant woman who smokes carries not only her own genetic burden but potentially imparts a genetic legacy of vulnerability to her offspring.

In this narrative, pregnant women stand at the precipice of profound decision-making. They bear the weight of responsibility not only for their own health but for the genetic well-being of their unborn children. The act of quitting smoking during pregnancy becomes an act of genetic guardianship—a choice that can potentially alter the trajectory of a family's genetic history.

It is a testament to the interconnectedness of life—a reminder that our choices have consequences that ripple through the delicate threads of DNA, affecting not only our own well-being but that of generations yet to come. Smoking, once seen as a solitary indulgence, emerges as a stark reminder of the collective genetic responsibility we bear—a responsibility to safeguard the integrity of our genetic legacy.

In conclusion, the impact of smoking extends far beyond its immediate health consequences, reaching into the very core of our genetic identity. Pregnant women who smoke not only jeopardize their own health but also risk altering the genetic destiny of their unborn children. The insidious effects of smoking on DNA, particularly through DNA methylation, can disrupt normal development and predispose children to a host of health issues. Furthermore, these genetic changes have the potential to be inherited, affecting future generations. Thus, the act of quitting smoking during pregnancy becomes a profound choice—a choice that can potentially rewrite the genetic narrative and protect the genetic legacy of generations to come.

Drugs

In the field of medicine, there exists a prevailing wisdom that is oftentimes overshadowed by the allure of pharmaceutical interventions—a wisdom encapsulated in the profound statement, "Drugs never cure disease, they just change the form and location of a disease." These words, though concise, carry within them the weight of a fundamental truth that has the power to reshape our understanding of health and healing.

Understanding this profound truth requires us to embark on an explorative journey, delving into the complex relationship between our physical bodies and the illnesses that impact us. This journey goes beyond merely observing the outward symptoms of disease, diving into the depths of our cellular and molecular makeup, where the intricate struggle between wellness and illness takes place. At the heart of this understanding lies a fundamental principle—that our bodies possess an innate ability to heal. This remarkable capacity for self-healing is not a mere theoretical concept; it is a tangible reality woven into the fabric of our existence. Within the intricate dance of cells and tissues, our bodies orchestrate a symphony of responses aimed at restoring equilibrium and vitality.

Yet, this inherent healing potential is often overshadowed by the allure of pharmaceutical drugs. In the pursuit of quick fixes and immediate relief, we turn to medications that promise to alleviate our symptoms and provide respite from discomfort. These drugs, while effective in their own right, carry with them a crucial distinction—they do not cure the underlying disease.

Instead, they function as agents of modification, altering the course of illness by changing its form and location within the body. This transformative process may bring temporary relief and offer a semblance of control over the disease, but it does not address the root cause. The disease may retreat to the shadows, only to resurface in a different guise or manifest in a different part of the body.

It is in this context that the story of a courageous woman with tumors in her abdomen unfolds—a story that serves as a beacon of hope and a testament to the transformative power of lifestyle and dietary choices. Faced with a daunting diagnosis, this woman made a remarkable decision—one that would challenge the conventional paradigm of disease treatment.

Rather than embarking on the arduous path of chemotherapy, with its accompanying side effects and uncertain outcomes, she chose a different route. She embarked on a specific diet and treatment plan—one designed to starve the cancer cells and alkalize her body. It was a choice rooted in the belief that the body's innate healing mechanisms could be harnessed and amplified through mindful dietary and lifestyle modifications.

The results of this decision were nothing short of astounding. As she adhered to her tailored regimen, the tumors that had once taken root in her abdomen began to recede. Slowly but steadily, her body responded to the nourishing effects of her chosen diet, and the cancer cells found themselves deprived of the sustenance they needed to thrive.

In time, the tumors disappeared entirely—a development that left her doctors incredulous. They bore witness to a transformation that defied conventional medical expectations. Not only had the tumors vanished, but her overall health had also improved dramatically. It was a testament to the power of holistic healing—an affirmation that the body, when provided with the right conditions, can start a self-restoration process.

The implications of this remarkable process reverberate far beyond the individual. They challenge the prevailing notion that disease is an insurmountable adversary best subdued by pharmaceutical interventions. Instead, they beckon us to explore the untapped potential of our bodies—the potential to heal, regenerate, and thrive.

In the narrative of this woman's triumph over tumors, we find a profound message—that the choices we make regarding our diets and lifestyles can wield a transformative influence on our health. These choices have the power to not only alleviate the symptoms of disease but to address its root causes. They enable us to engage with our bodies as active participants in the healing process, rather than passive recipients of medical interventions.

The story serves as a reminder that healing is not confined to the pharmaceutical sector only. It is a multifaceted experience that encompasses the nourishment of body and soul. It invites us to reconsider our approach to health and disease, to explore the potential of dietary and lifestyle modifications, and to acknowledge the profound truth that "Drugs never cure disease, they just change the form and location of a disease."

In the pages of this narrative, we find not only inspiration but also a call to action—a call to embrace the wisdom of holistic healing and to embark on a journey of self-discovery and transformation. It is a journey that transcends the boundaries of conventional medicine, leading us toward a profound understanding of the intricate dance between our bodies and the diseases we encounter along the way.

Sugar

In the landscape of modern dietary habits, one substance has emerged as both ubiquitous and insidious—an innocuous-looking crystal that goes by the name of sugar. It is a substance that has woven itself into the fabric of our lives, gracing our tables, sweetening our moments, and, quite often, wreaking havoc within our bodies. Sugar, in its various forms, has become an integral part of our diets, finding its way into an astonishing array of foods and beverages. Yet, beneath its sweet facade lies a truth that cannot be ignored—it has the ability to tamper with our very DNA.

The link between sugar and its deleterious effects on health has become increasingly apparent in recent years. One of the most alarming consequences of sugar abuse is its intimate connection to the global epidemic of diabetes—a condition that affects millions and places an enormous burden on healthcare systems worldwide. To understand this connection, we must delve into the intricate dance that sugar orchestrates within our bodies.

At its core, diabetes is a metabolic disorder characterized by elevated blood sugar levels, often resulting from the body's inability to properly utilize insulin, a hormone that regulates glucose uptake by cells. Herein lies the crux of the matter—sugar abuse can lead to diabetes by setting in motion a chain of events that culminates in elevated blood sugar levels and places tremendous strain on the pancreas, the organ responsible for producing insulin.

The journey begins with the consumption of sugar-rich foods and beverages, which flood the bloodstream with a surge of glucose—a form of sugar. This rapid influx of glucose triggers a spike in blood sugar levels, creating a state of imbalance within the body. In response to this surge, the pancreas springs into action, secreting insulin in an attempt to usher glucose into the cells, where it can be utilized for energy. It is a delicate and intricate process, finely tuned to maintain blood sugar levels within a narrow, optimal range.

However, sugar abuse disrupts this delicate equilibrium. The frequent and excessive consumption of sugary foods and drinks bombards the pancreas with an unrelenting demand for insulin. Over time, this unceasing demand can lead to a state of insulin resistance—an insidious condition in which the body's cells become less responsive to the hormone's signals. This resistance effectively locks the doors of the cells, preventing glucose from entering, and causing blood sugar levels to remain elevated.

The consequences of this relentless cycle are far-reaching and profound. Elevated blood sugar levels, if left unchecked, can inflict damage throughout the body. They can impair blood vessels, leading to cardiovascular complications, and they can wreak havoc on the delicate nerves of the nervous system, resulting in neuropathic disorders. Furthermore, sustained high blood sugar levels can exact a toll on the kidneys, potentially culminating in renal dysfunction.

Yet, the impact of sugar abuse extends beyond these immediate health concerns. Recent research has unveiled a disturbing truth—sugar has the ability to tamper with our genetic code, leaving a lasting imprint on our DNA.

In the intricate dance between sugar and DNA, a process known as glycation emerges as a central player. Glycation occurs when sugar molecules bind to proteins, lipids, or nucleic acids in the body, forming complex structures known as advanced glycation end-products (AGEs). These AGEs have the potential to inflict damage on various cellular components, including our precious DNA.

The consequences of DNA glycation are multifaceted and troubling. It can lead to a disruption in the structure and function of DNA, impairing its ability to carry out vital genetic instructions. This disruption can cascade into a myriad of health issues, potentially contributing to the development of chronic diseases.

Furthermore, the insidious effects of sugar on DNA extend beyond our own bodies. Recent studies have suggested that the dietary choices we make today may influence the health of future generations. The epigenetic modifications induced by sugar abuse can potentially be inherited by offspring, altering their genetic predisposition to various health conditions. It is a sobering realization—one that underscores the far-reaching impact of dietary choices on our genetic legacy.

In conclusion, the link between sugar and the global epidemic of diabetes is undeniable. Sugar abuse, with its ability to elevate blood sugar levels and strain the pancreas, plays a pivotal role in the development of this metabolic disorder. Yet, the story goes deeper, venturing into the universe of our DNA. Sugar's capacity to tamper with our genetic code through glycation is a stark reminder of the profound impact our dietary choices can have on our health. As we navigate the intricate relationship between sugar and our biology, we are compelled to reevaluate our consumption of this sweet seductress, recognizing that the consequences extend far beyond the palate and into the very fabric of our genetic heritage.

Q&A

1. What are the primary theories regarding the origin of diseases in the field of medicine?

— In the territory of medical theories, two prominent perspectives emerge: the innate healing prowess of the human body and the imperative comprehension of cellular and DNA mechanisms as contributors to disease onset.

2. How does lifestyle exert its influence on the emergence of diseases?

— The domain of epigenetics, as a compelling illustration, underscores the sway of lifestyle factors in shaping disease etiology, intertwining with genetic predispositions.

3. In what manner does our DNA exert control over the rejuvenation of cells?

— Within our DNA resides the blueprint for cell regeneration, with the nutrients sourced from our dietary choices actively participating in the perpetual cycle of cellular renewal within our organism.

4. Is it justifiable to attribute diseases solely to genetic factors?

— No, ascribing diseases exclusively to genetic origins absolves individuals of their personal responsibility for health, acknowledging the substantial role that lifestyle choices play in disease manifestation.

5. What factors can instigate mineral deficiencies in the human body?

— The genesis of mineral deficiencies in our bodies can be traced to multifarious factors, encompassing agricultural practices that deplete minerals from the soil and the erosive impact of stimulants like sugar and caffeine, which leach essential minerals from our corporeal reservoirs.

Chapter 2: Nutrition and Diet

There exists a profound axiom—an axiom that echoes through the corridors of time, resonating with wisdom and insight. It is a statement uttered by the ancient Greek physician Hippocrates, a figure whose contributions to the field of medicine remain legendary to this day. "Let food be your medicine and medicine be your food," declared Hippocrates, encapsulating a philosophy that transcends generations and cultures.

Within these words lies a profound revelation—an invitation to explore the intricate relationship between nutrition and the fundamental building blocks of life itself—our DNA. In the tapestry of our existence, the DNA molecule stands as a blueprint, a genetic code that orchestrates the symphony of life within each of our cells. It is a code that holds the secrets of our uniqueness, our health, and our destiny.

As we delve into the depths of this wisdom, we are beckoned to contemplate the pivotal role that nutrition plays in maintaining the integrity of our DNA. The foods we choose to nourish our bodies are not merely sustenance; they are the raw materials from which our DNA draws its strength and resilience. Just as a master builder selects the finest bricks and mortar for a grand edifice, so too must we choose our foods with care and mindfulness.

In embracing the philosophy of "food as medicine," we recognize that our dietary choices are not separate from our well-being; they are intrinsic to it. The foods we consume carry the potential to either fortify our DNA, empowering it to withstand the tests of time, or to undermine its integrity, paving the way for health challenges. It is a profound responsibility, one that places the power of health and vitality firmly within our hands.

Hippocrates' wisdom extends further, casting light upon the intricate relationship between gut health and overall well-being. "All disease begins in the gut," proclaimed this ancient sage, a statement that reverberates through the annals of medical history. In these words, we find a profound acknowledgment of the gut's central role in the tapestry of health—a role that extends far beyond digestion.

The gut, often regarded as the seat of our immune system, is a bustling ecosystem teeming with microorganisms—bacteria, viruses, fungi, and more. These microscopic inhabitants, collectively known as the gut microbiome, play a pivotal role in our health. They are the guardians of our gastrointestinal tract, maintaining a delicate balance between health and disease.

When we contemplate Hippocrates' assertion that "all disease begins in the gut," we are prompted to delve into the intricate web of connections that link gut health to various health conditions. The gut microbiome, influenced by our dietary choices and lifestyle, exerts a profound influence on our immune system, inflammation, and even our mental well-being. The choices we make ripple through the fabric of our health, shaping our susceptibility to diseases and our ability to thrive.

When we consider our diet, we find a formidable partner—a force that enhances the robustness of our DNA and the wellness of our digestive system. This path begins with conscious decisions made at every meal, transforming each dish into a chance to internally strengthen ourselves. The food we choose, laden with vital nutrients, antioxidants, and phytonutrients, transcends basic caloric value; these are the cornerstones of our wellbeing.

The concept of "food as medicine" leads us on an exploration into the realm of natural, unprocessed foods—embracing fruits, vegetables, grains, nuts, and seeds. It's a journey about delighting in nature's array of flavors, enjoying the rich colors of various fruits and vegetables, and harnessing the healing power of herbs and spices. On this path, we reconnect with the age-old wisdom of traditional diets and uncover the therapeutic benefits of plant-based eating.

However, the road to optimal health isn't limited to nutrition. It also involves caring for our digestive health, fostering a thriving gut microbiome that underpins our overall wellbeing. Foods rich in probiotics, like yogurt, kefir, sauerkraut, and kimchi, become valuable tools in this pursuit. They enrich our digestive system with beneficial bacteria, bolstering our immune system and promoting a balanced and harmonious state.

In our health's vast landscape, the interaction among nutrition, DNA, and gut health plays out like a symphony, where every choice contributes to our overall wellbeing's harmony. Following Hippocrates' wisdom, we embark on a path of empowerment, shaping our health destiny.

In essence, Hippocrates' timeless wisdom continues to echo, inviting us to acknowledge the deep link between our diet, genetic health, and gut wellness. His famous adage, "Let food be your medicine and medicine be your food," remains a powerful testament to the significant influence our dietary habits have on our genetic integrity. Similarly, his assertion that "all disease begins in the gut" highlights the crucial role of gut health in our overall wellbeing. This journey is one of self-discovery and empowerment, where each meal is an opportunity to nourish our health and vitality.

The Philosophy of Wholesome Eating

Dr. O'Neill transcends the mere act of eating and ventures where food becomes a conduit for healing, vitality, and connection. Wholesome eating, a cornerstone of this enlightening journey, emerges not only as a nutritional choice but as a holistic approach to living. Within this domain, I, as a devoted researcher and follower of the teachings that have shaped countless lives towards better health, share reflections and insights gleaned from a journey deeply rooted in the wisdom of nature and the guidance of a seasoned mentor in the field of holistic health.

The essence of wholesome eating, as championed in our journey, goes beyond the conventional understanding of nutrition. It's a philosophy that views food as an integral part of the larger tapestry of life, interwoven with our physical, emotional, and spiritual well-being. This understanding has been a guiding light in my own exploration, transforming my relationship with food from one of mere sustenance to a deeper, more meaningful interaction. I've learned that the choices we make at the dinner table are not just about pleasing our palates but about nourishing our bodies at the cellular level, nurturing our souls, and respecting the intricate balance of the natural world.

In practicing this philosophy, I have experienced firsthand the transformative power of a diet that prioritizes whole, unprocessed foods. This shift towards a more natural, plant-centered diet was not just a change in eating habits but a profound awakening to the intricacies of our biological needs. It's about understanding the innate wisdom of our bodies and the subtle ways they communicate their needs. As someone who has walked the path from processed to whole foods, I have witnessed remarkable changes, not just in physical health but in mental clarity and emotional balance.

Additionally, the concept of wholesome eating extends its reach beyond individual health, underscoring the interconnected nature of our world. This comprehensive viewpoint prompts us to reflect on the origins of our food, tracing its path from the initial seed to our dining tables, and to acknowledge the effects our dietary decisions have on both the environment and global communities. As a researcher delving into the intricacies of sustainable farming and ethical sourcing, I've developed a profound respect for the fragile equilibrium that upholds our earth.

In this exploration, the kitchen has transformed into a haven for healing and creativity. It's a place where the magic of mixing natural ingredients results in meals that are not just nourishing, but also restorative. This approach to cooking and meal preparation, rooted in the wisdom of our teachings, is akin to an art form. In this art, each ingredient is selected with purpose, and every dish is crafted with attentiveness and appreciation.

Moreover, the concept of wholesome eating is dynamic, continuously evolving alongside us. It represents a deeply personal journey, one that explores what truly nourishes each individual, acknowledging the uniqueness of everyone's route to health. This tailored approach has been a crucial takeaway from my studies and practice, constantly reminding me that nutrition is not a one-size-fits-all discipline.

The concept of wholesome eating, integral to holistic nutrition, represents a return to the fundamentals of true nourishment. This approach beckons us to delve into a deeper understanding of health, to forge a stronger bond with nature, and to live in a manner that respects the intricate connection between our well-being, our diet, and the planet. As a contributor to this philosophy, I offer these insights with the aspiration of inspiring others to commence their explorations and transformations.

Embedded within this philosophy, which has guided countless individuals towards enriched well-being, lies a profound understanding of our interconnectedness with the natural environment. This viewpoint not only sustains our physical bodies but also enriches our souls and minds, fostering a balance that is in tune with the earth's natural rhythms. My role as a dedicated learner and investigator in this field has been a journey marked by significant growth and introspection, guided by the principles of holistic wellness.

In embracing this philosophy, one of the most significant revelations has been the understanding of food as a powerful agent of change. Each dietary choice we make can be a step towards healing, a gesture of respect towards our environment, and a contribution to our overall well-being. This perspective shift was not an overnight transformation but a gradual awakening to the intricate web of life where our food choices play a pivotal role. The realization that what we eat directly impacts our health, mood, and energy levels was both empowering and humbling. It bestowed upon me a sense of responsibility to make informed, conscious choices, not just for my health but for the well-being of the planet.

The principles of wholesome eating advocate for a diet that is rich in natural, unrefined foods – a celebration of the bounty that nature offers in its purest form. My personal transition to this way of eating was marked by an exploration of a variety of whole grains, legumes, nuts, seeds, fruits, and vegetables, each bursting with flavors, textures, and colors. This was not merely a dietary change but an exploration of the vast palette of nature's offerings. The experience of tasting foods in their most natural state, free from heavy processing and artificial additives, was like rediscovering the authentic tastes and aromas that had been masked in my previous diet of processed foods.

Moreover, this journey brought with it an appreciation for the art of cooking from scratch, where each ingredient is chosen for its nutritional value and its contribution to the overall harmony of the dish. Cooking became a meditative practice, a time to connect with the ingredients, understanding their origins, and the effort that went into growing them.

This connection brought a newfound respect for food and the farmers who cultivate it, underscoring the importance of supporting sustainable and ethical farming practices.

Incorporating the wisdom of herbalism into this philosophy further enriched my understanding of food as medicine. Herbs and spices, once mere flavor enhancers, became vital components of my diet for their health-promoting properties. Learning about the healing properties of herbs like turmeric, ginger, basil, and many others, and incorporating them into daily meals, opened up a world of natural remedies that support health and prevent illness.

This approach also underscores the significance of attuning to our body's needs and deciphering its signals. Throughout my own experience, I have become adept at recognizing my body's indications of hunger and satiety, its requirements for specific nutrients, and the kinds of nourishment that optimally support my well-being in varying circumstances. This form of intuitive eating, informed by a holistic understanding of nutrition, has reshaped my relationship with food from a paradigm of limitations and regulations to one centered on sustenance and pleasure.

Embarking on the path of embracing wholesome eating is an ongoing process, replete with discovery, experimentation, and personal growth. It's a journey that calls for patience, openness, and an eagerness to adapt to new ideas. By sharing these insights and experiences, I aspire to encourage others to venture down this rewarding path. This journey involves uncovering the delight and wellness found in aligning with the natural rhythms of our diets and adopting a lifestyle that fosters both personal and global well-being. It transcends mere dietary habits; it's about leading a life that harmonizes with nature, promoting health and balance.

The Power of a Plant-Based Diet

Exploring Barbara's suggestions about holistic nutrition, I noticed that a profound emphasis is placed on the power of a plant-based diet, a concept that resonates deeply with the teachings I have embraced and shared. This philosophy isn't just a dietary choice but a comprehensive approach to health that is backed by an array of scientific findings. Understanding the reasons behind the efficacy of a plant-based diet reveals the harmony between our body's natural processes and the nutrients provided by the earth.

From a scientific standpoint, the emphasis on whole foods in a plant-based diet is crucial. These foods are in their most natural state, unstripped of essential nutrients that are often lost in processing. Whole foods provide a wealth of essential nutrients in a form that the body recognizes and can utilize efficiently. For instance, the complex carbohydrates in whole plant foods offer a steady source of energy, unlike refined sugars which can lead to energy spikes and crashes. Additionally, the fiber present in whole foods not only aids digestion but also plays a significant role in regulating blood sugar and cholesterol levels, contributing to overall heart health.

Plant-based diets are inherently rich in a variety of nutrients essential for optimal health. They are packed with vitamins, minerals, antioxidants, and phytonutrients that work synergistically to support the body's functions and protect against disease. Scientific research has shown that the antioxidants found in plant foods can reduce oxidative stress, a contributor to aging and chronic diseases. Furthermore, the diverse range of phytonutrients, each with unique benefits, contribute to the prevention and management of various health conditions. For instance, flavonoids found in berries and leafy greens have been linked to improved cognitive function and reduced inflammation.

The role of a plant-based diet in preventing and managing chronic diseases is well-documented. Scientific studies have consistently shown that populations consuming diets rich in fruits, vegetables, and whole grains have lower rates of heart disease, diabetes, and certain types of cancer. This protective effect is attributed to the low levels of harmful fats and high levels of dietary fiber and essential nutrients in plant-based foods. For example, the fiber in plant foods not only helps in regulating digestion but also plays a role in cancer prevention, particularly in the gastrointestinal tract.

Adopting a plant-based diet often results in increased energy levels and overall well-being. This is because plant foods provide sustained energy through their complex carbohydrates and essential nutrients. These foods support metabolic processes and contribute to the optimal functioning of various bodily systems. Many individuals who transition to a plant-based diet report improvements in vitality, mood, and mental clarity, highlighting the diet's positive impact on overall quality of life.

The environmental and ethical implications of a plant-based diet are also significant. From a sustainability perspective, plant-based diets require fewer resources such as water and land, and they have a lower environmental impact compared to diets high in animal products. This aspect aligns with the holistic principle of living in harmony with nature and taking responsibility for the health of our planet.

In summary, from the perspective of holistic nutrition, a plant-based diet is not only beneficial for individual health but also for the well-being of our environment. The scientific evidence supporting this approach to eating highlights the interconnectedness of our diet, our health, and the world we live in. Embracing a plant-based diet is therefore a step towards a more holistic, healthful, and sustainable way of living.

Understanding Macronutrients and Micronutrients

In the exploration of a balanced diet, a crucial element lies in comprehending the intricate dance between macronutrients and micronutrients, a dance that is fundamental to sustaining life and promoting health. As a researcher who has delved deeply into the teachings of holistic nutrition, I have come to appreciate the delicate balance and the profound importance of these nutritional components in our daily diet. This understanding is not just a matter of scientific knowledge, but a profound insight into the way our bodies function and thrive.

Macronutrients, comprising carbohydrates, proteins, and fats, are the pillars of our diet, each playing a unique and vital role in maintaining our health. Carbohydrates, often misunderstood and sometimes unfairly maligned in popular diet culture, are in fact the body's primary source of energy. They fuel our brain, our muscles, and are essential for the functioning of our internal organs. The key, as I have learned through both study and personal experience, lies in choosing the right types of carbohydrates – those that are unrefined and rich in fiber, such as whole grains, fruits, and vegetables, which provide sustained energy and support digestive health.

Proteins, the building blocks of our body, are crucial for the repair and growth of tissues. They play a critical role in the formation of enzymes and hormones and are essential for maintaining muscle mass and overall metabolic health. My journey in the world of herbalism has shown me that proteins are not just confined to animal sources; a myriad of plant-based options like legumes, nuts, and seeds are excellent sources of protein and are accompanied by an array of other health-promoting nutrients.

Fats, often the subject of much debate, are in fact an essential component of a healthy diet. They are vital for the absorption of fat-soluble vitamins and for the health of our cells, including our brain cells. The focus, however, should be on consuming healthy fats found in foods like avocados, nuts, seeds, and certain oils, which support heart health and reduce inflammation, rather than on the saturated and trans fats that can contribute to health problems.

The role of micronutrients, which includes vitamins and minerals, though required in smaller quantities, is no less significant. These nutrients are involved in virtually every process within the body. Vitamins such as Vitamin C, essential for immune function, and Vitamin D, crucial for bone health, are just a few examples of the myriad of functions these nutrients support. Minerals like calcium, necessary for strong bones and teeth, and iron, essential for transporting oxygen in the blood, highlight the diverse roles micronutrients play in our health.

The understanding macronutrients and micronutrients is not something just academic; it is a practical guide to how we should approach our diet. It teaches us that a balanced diet is not about rigid restrictions or following the latest diet trends. Rather, it's about creating a harmonious plate that supports our body's needs. It's about choosing a variety of foods, in their most natural form, to ensure we are getting the right balance of nutrients. This approach to eating is not only nourishing but also sustainable and aligned with the principles of holistic health.

In conclusion, the essentials of a balanced diet, rooted in the understanding of macronutrients and micronutrients, form the foundation of good health. It is a testament to the wisdom of nature, which provides us with everything we need to thrive. As we continue our exploration into the world of holistic nutrition, this understanding becomes a guiding light, illuminating the path towards a healthier, more vibrant life.

The Importance of Whole Foods

Following Barbara's teachings about a balanced diet, I reveal the profound importance of whole foods, not merely as elements of our diet but as the very core of nourishing both body and spirit. As an herbalist and researcher influenced by holistic principles that emphasize the benefits of natural, unrefined foods, I've grown to understand and champion the critical role of whole foods in our well-being. This understanding is rooted in the recognition that whole foods, in their purest form, deliver a rich tapestry of nutrients, tastes, and vital properties, often diminished in processed alternatives.

Pursuing a diet centered around whole foods is as much an exploration of nature's bountiful produce as it is a journey to understand how these foods interact with our physiology. Foods in their whole state, abundant in vitamins, minerals, fiber, and a spectrum of phytonutrients, synergistically nourish and defend our bodies. Consider the simple example of eating a fresh apple, complete with its fiber-rich skin and antioxidants, compared to consuming a processed apple product where these valuable components are typically reduced. The whole apple is not just nutritionally beneficial but also embodies the principle of consuming foods as nature provides them.

In my research and personal practice, transitioning to a diet rich in whole foods has been a journey of transformation. I've observed the profound impact of this change on health, both in myself and others. The shift leads to improved digestive health due to the high fiber content of whole foods and boosts immune function through an array of vitamins and antioxidants. Furthermore, whole foods are instrumental in managing and preventing chronic diseases. The natural compounds found in these foods, like the heart-healthy fats in nuts and seeds or the anti-inflammatory properties of leafy greens, contribute to a comprehensive approach to wellness that views the body as an interconnected system.

Choosing whole foods also transcends personal health, touching upon environmental sustainability and conscious consumption. These foods, in their unprocessed state, typically require fewer resources for production and processing than refined foods. Opting for whole foods is a decision that benefits personal health and supports a more sustainable and ethical food system, an increasingly crucial aspect in today's global context.

Incorporating whole foods into one's diet is an adventure in culinary creativity. It encourages the preparation of meals that are not just healthful but also diverse and flavorful. Cooking with whole ingredients is a gratifying experience, fostering a connection to our food sources and a sense of fulfillment from knowing that what we eat is beneficial for both our bodies and the planet.

In conclusion, the importance of whole foods in a balanced diet cannot be overstated. They are the foundation upon which good health is built, offering a wealth of nutritional benefits and supporting a lifestyle that is in harmony with nature. As we delve deeper into the principles of holistic nutrition, the role of whole foods stands out as a key element, guiding us towards a way of eating and living that is nourishing, sustainable, and deeply fulfilling.

Barbara O'Neill often recommends various whole foods, emphasizing their natural health benefits. Here's a list of some whole foods she suggests and the reasons why they are beneficial:

Leafy Greens (e.g., spinach, kale, Swiss chard): These are high in vitamins A, C, E, and K, and contain abundant minerals like calcium and iron. They are also rich in fiber and phytonutrients, which are known for their anti-inflammatory and antioxidant properties.

Berries (e.g., blueberries, strawberries, raspberries): Berries are packed with antioxidants, particularly anthocyanins, which may reduce the risk of chronic diseases and aid in maintaining cognitive function. They are also high in fiber and vitamin C.

Nuts and Seeds (e.g., almonds, flaxseeds, chia seeds): These are excellent sources of healthy fats, including omega-3 fatty acids, vital for heart health. They also provide protein, fiber, and important minerals like magnesium and zinc.

Whole Grains (e.g., quinoa, brown rice, oats): Whole grains are important sources of fiber, B vitamins, and minerals such as iron, magnesium, and selenium. The fiber in whole grains helps with digestive health and can aid in the prevention of cardiovascular diseases.

Legumes (e.g., lentils, chickpeas, black beans): Legumes are a great source of plant-based protein, fiber, and various nutrients. They can aid in regulating blood sugar levels, improving cholesterol levels, and supporting digestive health.

Root Vegetables (e.g., sweet potatoes, carrots, beets): These are high in fiber, vitamins, and minerals. For instance, sweet potatoes are rich in beta-carotene, which is beneficial for eye health and the immune system.

Cruciferous Vegetables (e.g., broccoli, cauliflower, Brussels sprouts): Known for their cancer-fighting properties, these vegetables are rich in fiber, vitamins C, E, K, and folate, and contain glucosinolates, which have been shown to have anti-cancer effects.

Fruits (e.g., apples, oranges, bananas): Fruits are high in vitamins, minerals, fiber, and antioxidants. They offer a wide range of health benefits, from improving digestion to reducing the risk of chronic diseases.

Fermented Foods (e.g., sauerkraut, kimchi, natural yogurt): These foods are beneficial for gut health due to their probiotic content. They help in maintaining a healthy balance of gut flora, which is crucial for digestion, immunity, and even mental health.

Avocados: Rich in monounsaturated fats, which are heart-healthy, avocados also provide fiber and essential nutrients like potassium.

Barbara O'Neill's emphasis on these whole foods is based on their natural composition, which is in harmony with the body's nutritional needs. Consuming these foods in their whole, unprocessed form maximizes the intake of essential nutrients that are often lost during processing. This approach to diet is reflective of her philosophy on natural health and preventive care through nutrition.

In the intricate tapestry of holistic health, the philosophy of using nutrition for health and healing stands as a testament to the power of natural foods in both preventing and treating various health conditions. As a researcher and practitioner deeply influenced by the teachings that advocate for this approach, I have come to understand and appreciate the profound role diet plays in influencing our health. This exploration delves into the ways in which specific dietary choices can prevent and even treat certain health conditions, aligning with the natural processes of our bodies for restoration and healing.

The concept of using food as medicine is ancient, yet it holds immense relevance in our modern world, where chronic diseases are prevalent. The foundation of this approach is the understanding that the right nutrients can not only nourish the body but also fortify it against illnesses. For instance, diets rich in fruits, vegetables, whole grains, and lean proteins are linked with lower incidences of chronic diseases such as heart disease, diabetes, and certain cancers. These foods, brimming with essential nutrients, antioxidants, and phytochemicals, play a crucial role in maintaining cellular health and preventing the onset of disease.

Disease/Condition	Recommended Foods	Healing Properties
Heart Disease	Omega-3 rich foods (flaxseeds, walnuts, fatty fish), whole grains, leafy greens (spinach, kale)	Reduce inflammation, improve cholesterol profiles, protect against heart disease
Cancer	Fruits and vegetables (especially rich in antioxidants), cruciferous vegetables (broccoli, Brussels sprouts), tomatoes	Protect cells from damage, reduce risk of certain cancers, support immune function
Digestive Health	High fiber foods, fermented foods (kefir, sauerkraut, kimchi), foods low in sugar and processed ingredients	Support digestive health, enhance gut flora, aid in nutrient absorption
Autoimmune and Inflammatory Conditions	Anti-inflammatory foods (ginger, turmeric, berries), omega-3 rich foods, reduction of refined sugars and processed foods	Reduce body inflammation, support immune function, alleviate symptoms of autoimmune conditions

Heart Disease and Diet

In addressing cardiovascular health, the emphasis is often placed on reducing intake of harmful fats and increasing consumption of heart-healthy nutrients. Foods rich in omega-3 fatty acids, such as flaxseeds, walnuts, and fatty fish like salmon, are highly recommended. These foods help in reducing inflammation and improving cholesterol profiles. Additionally, the incorporation of whole grains into the diet contributes to cardiovascular health. Whole grains provide essential fibers which aid in reducing blood pressure and improving heart health. The integration of a variety of fruits and vegetables, especially those high in antioxidants, can further fortify the heart against disease. For instance, leafy greens like spinach and kale are lauded for their vitamin K content, crucial for heart health.

Cancer Prevention and Nutrition

If we talk about cancer prevention, a diet rich in fruits and vegetables is often highlighted for its potential to reduce cancer risk. These foods are packed with antioxidants and phytochemicals that protect cells from damage. For example, the lycopene found in tomatoes has been linked to a reduced risk of prostate cancer. Similarly, cruciferous vegetables like broccoli and Brussels sprouts contain sulforaphane, a compound with potent anti-cancer properties. The emphasis is also on reducing the intake of processed and red meats, which have been linked to an increased risk of certain cancers.

Gut Health and Dietary Choices

The health of the digestive system is paramount in holistic health paradigms. A diet high in fiber is crucial for maintaining gut health. Fiber not only aids digestion but also acts as a prebiotic, feeding beneficial gut bacteria. Fermented foods, rich in probiotics, like kefir, sauerkraut, and kimchi, are often recommended to enhance gut flora. These beneficial bacteria play a significant role in nutrient absorption, immune function, and even mental health. Avoiding foods that irritate the gut lining, such as excessive sugar and processed foods, is also a key aspect of maintaining digestive health.

Autoimmune and Inflammatory Conditions

For those dealing with autoimmune and inflammatory conditions, dietary adjustments can be a powerful tool. Anti-inflammatory foods like ginger, turmeric, and berries are often recommended. These foods contain compounds that help reduce inflammation in the body. Additionally, the elimination or reduction of inflammatory foods, such as refined sugars and processed foods, is advised. The inclusion of healthy fats, particularly those rich in omega-3 fatty acids, is also emphasized due to their anti-inflammatory properties.

Implementing Nutritional Changes

Barbara O'Neill, known for her holistic approach to health and nutrition, suggests several key principles when it comes to implementing nutritional changes and transitioning to a healthier diet. These principles are rooted in her belief in the healing power of natural foods and the importance of lifestyle changes for overall health and well-being. Here's an overview of her approach:

Start with Gradual Changes: O'Neill often emphasizes the importance of making gradual dietary changes rather than abrupt shifts. This could mean starting by incorporating more fruits and vegetables into one's diet, gradually reducing processed foods, or slowly introducing whole grains and legumes. The idea is to allow the body and palate to adjust to these changes over time.

Hydration and Natural Foods: O'Neill often discusses the importance of hydration and the consumption of foods in their most natural state. Drinking sufficient water and consuming fresh, unprocessed foods can significantly improve health and aid in the prevention of diseases.

Listen to Your Body: She advocates listening to your body's signals. This involves understanding and responding to your body's hunger cues and recognizing how different foods affect your mood, energy levels, and overall health.

Balance and Moderation: O'Neill encourages a balanced approach to eating. This means consuming a variety of foods to ensure a wide range of nutrients and practicing moderation, even with healthy foods, to maintain a balanced diet.

Educate Yourself about Nutrition: O'Neill stresses the importance of education in nutrition. Understanding what constitutes a healthy diet and the role of different nutrients can empower individuals to make informed food choices.

Incorporate Physical Activity: Alongside dietary changes, incorporating regular physical activity is a key part of her holistic approach to health. Exercise complements nutritional efforts, enhancing overall health and well-being.

Mindful Eating: She also talks about the importance of mindful eating – being present and attentive during meals, which can lead to a more enjoyable and satisfying eating experience.

In her teachings, Barbara O'Neill advocates for a holistic view of health where dietary changes are part of a larger lifestyle approach. This includes not just what we eat but how we eat and how we live our lives, emphasizing the connection between diet, lifestyle, and overall health.

In pursuing better health and wellness, transitioning to a more nutritious diet emerges as a crucial step, a voyage characterized by both its challenges and significant rewards. Immersed in the world of holistic nutrition and herbal medicine, I have grown to understand and value the nuanced and intricate process of adopting enduring dietary changes. This path, often driven by the desire to embrace foods that naturally enhance health, is about reshaping one's relationship with food just as much as it is about altering food choices.

Beginning this journey typically involves a fundamental shift in how we perceive food. It's about seeing our meals not just as sources of fleeting enjoyment or convenience but as integral to sustained health and energy. This change in mindset is a vital initial move, setting the foundation for the tangible dietary adjustments that follow. In my experience and through assisting others, I've noticed that this change in attitude towards food and health usually springs from an epiphany – a recognition of the deep influence our diet has on our overall well-being and life quality.

The practicalities of transitioning to a healthier diet involve more than just choosing different foods; it requires a holistic approach. It begins with an understanding of one's current eating habits and identifying areas for improvement. This self-reflection is crucial, as it allows for a tailored approach to dietary change. For some, it might mean reducing the intake of processed foods and sugars, while for others, it might involve incorporating more fruits and vegetables or exploring plant-based protein sources. The key is to start with small, manageable changes, allowing the body and palate time to adjust.

One of the most significant challenges in this transition is overcoming reliance on processed and convenience foods. These foods, often high in unhealthy fats, sugars, and artificial additives, are designed to be highly palatable, making them difficult to resist. Breaking this pattern requires a conscious effort to seek out whole, natural foods and to rediscover the intrinsic flavors and textures that they offer. The experience of savoring a freshly prepared meal made with whole, unprocessed ingredients is not only more satisfying but also nourishing on a deeper level.

Cooking plays a central role in this transition. It is through the act of preparing meals that one can truly connect with the food, understanding its origin and the nourishment it provides. Cooking from scratch might seem daunting at first, especially for those who are not accustomed to it, but it becomes an empowering practice, a way to take control of one's health. It also opens up a world of culinary exploration, allowing one to experiment with new ingredients, flavors, and cooking techniques.

Another aspect of implementing nutritional changes is education. Understanding the nutritional value of different foods and how they affect the body is crucial. This knowledge not only guides better food choices but also fosters a deeper appreciation for the role of nutrition in health. In my research and practice, I have always emphasized the importance of continuous learning – exploring the latest findings in nutritional science and understanding traditional wisdom about food and health.

Social and emotional factors also play a significant role in transitioning to a healthier diet. Food is often intertwined with social interactions, cultural traditions, and emotional experiences. Navigating these aspects requires a balanced approach, one that allows for flexibility and mindfulness. It's about making conscious choices without depriving oneself of the joy and social aspects of eating. Sharing healthy meals with family and friends, for instance, can make the transition more enjoyable and sustainable.

In conclusion, transitioning to a healthier diet is a process that encompasses a range of physical, emotional, and social elements. It's a path of discovery, learning, and growth, leading to a more harmonious relationship with food and health. As one progresses along this path, the initial challenges give way to a newfound sense of vitality and well-being, a testament to the power of nutritional changes.

Weight Loss

Understanding weight loss involves a deep dive into the impact of diet, a factor that cannot be overlooked. A prevalent issue in the modern diet is the high consumption of carbohydrates, often seen in everyday foods like bread and cereal, which contributes significantly to weight gain and triggers cravings for less nutritious options. This observation leads us to examine the roles of different macronutrients in our diets, especially when the objective is shedding excess weight.

In many weight loss diets, there's a common tendency to demonize fats and reduce their intake drastically. However, it's essential to acknowledge the role of fat in providing a sense of satiation and overall satisfaction. From an energy standpoint, calories are the unit of measurement, and fats are calorie-dense, offering nine calories per gram, over twice the energy yield of glucose at four calories per gram. This higher energy content means that fats can be more satisfying and maintain energy for extended periods, making them a crucial component in a balanced diet for effective weight loss.

Historically, certain fats like coconut oil and olive oil have been renowned for their health benefits, being integral parts of diets for centuries, particularly in regions like the South Pacific Islands. These oils have proven their worth over time, demonstrating their beneficial role in sustaining good health.

The introduction of highly processed and refined foods, often referred to as the 'white man's diet,' consisting of white sugar, white rice, white flour, refined salt, and cow's milk, has been linked to a rise in health issues. In areas like the South Pacific Islands, where diets traditionally included coconut oil, this shift led to increased cases of obesity, heart disease, and diabetes, highlighting the negative impact of such dietary changes.

Dr. Atkins was a forerunner in questioning established dietary beliefs, particularly the dangers of high carbohydrate diets. His approach, emphasizing the significance of a balanced diet that includes meat, butter, cream cheese, and eggs, led to remarkable health improvements in his patients. These improvements included cancer remission and normalized cholesterol levels, challenging the typical dietary recommendations.

For effective weight loss, adopting a diet low in carbohydrates, rich in fiber, abundant in protein, and inclusive of healthy fats, along with a higher water intake, can lead to significant and positive changes. This dietary strategy not only assists in weight management but also resonates with a holistic view of health, highlighting the necessity for a nutritious and balanced diet. By understanding the complex roles of various macronutrients and the history of dietary habits, individuals are empowered to make choices that support their health and weight loss objectives, avoiding the common pitfalls of fashionable diets that might be counterproductive.

In her insightful exploration of weight management and overall wellness, Barbara O'Neill sheds light on the remarkable benefits of High-Intensity Interval Training (HIIT) for weight loss. Her research delves into the ways in which this training method, requiring as little as 15 minutes a day, can lead to significant health improvements, including more effective weight management.

One of the foundational principles highlighted by O'Neill is the concept of time-restricted eating. This approach allows the stomach a much-needed break between meals, thereby enhancing the restoration of digestive enzymes. The result of this practice is not just improved digestion but also a notable contribution to weight loss efforts.

High-Intensity Interval Training stands out in O'Neill's work for its dramatic impact on weight loss. The beauty of HIIT lies in its efficiency – requiring only a brief daily commitment of 15 minutes. This form of exercise is not only manageable in terms of time but also remarkably effective in stimulating the body's natural processes that contribute to weight loss.

A key physiological response to high-intensity exercise, as O'Neill points out, is the release of human growth hormone. This hormone plays a crucial role in stimulating the breakdown of fat stores, turning the body into a more efficient fat burner. This process is a cornerstone in achieving and maintaining a healthy weight.

O'Neill also draws attention to the lesser-known benefits of HIIT, such as its impact on skin health and the aging process. It's an interesting observation that while movie stars might spend a thousand dollars a week to increase blood circulation to the skin, thereby slowing down the appearance of wrinkles and aging, similar benefits can be achieved through regular high-intensity interval training. This natural boost in blood circulation to the skin, achievable through just 15 minutes of HIIT, underscores the holistic benefits of this exercise method, extending beyond weight loss to encompass overall physical appearance and health.

Barbara O'Neill's insights into High-Intensity Interval Training reveal it as a multifaceted tool not only for effective weight management but also for enhancing digestive efficiency, promoting healthy aging, and improving skin health, all within a time-efficient and accessible daily routine.

In her comprehensive study on the path to weight loss, Barbara O'Neill emphasizes the profound role that mindset plays in this transformative process. Her research underscores the dynamic and adaptable nature of the human brain, offering a beacon of hope not just for those aiming to shed pounds but also for anyone seeking to enhance their sleep quality and overall well-being.

O'Neill brings to light the empowering realization that our brains have the remarkable ability to rewire themselves throughout our lives. This neuroplasticity suggests that the way we think, feel, and approach our health goals, including weight loss, can be reshaped and refined over time. This aspect is crucial, as it opens the door to adopting healthier habits and perspectives that are essential in the journey towards a healthier weight.

Furthermore, O'Neill stresses the importance of lifestyle in maintaining beauty and youthfulness. Her findings reveal that lifestyle choices often have a more significant impact than genetics in preserving a youthful appearance and vitality. This insight is particularly relevant for those focused on weight loss, as it highlights the broader benefits of lifestyle modifications that extend beyond mere aesthetics.

Central to O'Neill's thesis is the concept that the mind is a key factor in achieving weight loss and transforming the body. The way we think about ourselves, our health, and our ability to change plays a pivotal role in determining the success of our weight loss efforts. By fostering a positive, determined, and resilient mindset, individuals can significantly increase their chances of reaching their weight loss goals.

In essence, Barbara O'Neill's research paints a holistic picture of weight loss, where the power of the mind is just as critical as the physical aspects of diet and exercise. Her work inspires a comprehensive approach to weight management, where mental and emotional well-being are integral to achieving and sustaining a healthy body weight.

Q&A

Q: What primarily contributes to weight gain?

A: The primary contributor to weight gain is an excess intake of carbohydrates, particularly refined carbs like bread, cereal, and pasta. These foods lead to an overabundance of glucose, which is then stored in the body as fat.

Q: What are the key food groups to focus on for losing weight?

A: For effective weight loss, the focus should be on a diet that is low in carbohydrates but rich in fiber, protein, and healthy fats. Excessive consumption of non-essential carbohydrates is often linked to obesity and other health complications.

Q: Which exercise is most effective for losing weight?

A: High intensity interval training (HIIT) is highly recommended for weight loss. This involves cycles of high intensity exercise, such as 30 seconds of vigorous activity, followed by 90 seconds of recovery. This routine, which can be completed in just 15 minutes a day, significantly impacts weight loss.

Q: How does hormone balance affect weight loss?

A: Hormonal balance plays a vital role in weight loss. The discussion will include an exploration of symptoms indicating hormonal imbalances and strategies for restoring this balance, as such imbalances can impede weight loss efforts.

Q: What is the role of breathing in weight loss?

A: Breathing techniques are crucial for weight loss. Nasal breathing activates the parasympathetic nervous system, leading to a calmer state and more efficient oxygen absorption by the cells. In contrast, mouth breathing engages the sympathetic nervous system, increasing heart rate.

Bonus #1: Video Recipes

As you turn the pages of "Dr. Barbara Bible," immersing yourself in the profound teachings of Dr. Barbara O'Neill as artfully presented by Simon Jr. Jackson, I am excited to offer you a special invitation to further explore the realm of natural health.. Within this message lies a special QR code, a gateway to an exceptional bonus content meticulously aligned with Barbara's teachings on holistic wellness.

This QR code leads you to an exclusive collection of Anti-Inflammatory Video Recipes. These recipes are more than just culinary guides; they are a manifestation of Barbara's philosophy, blending her deep understanding of natural health with practical, everyday applications. Each video recipe is crafted to echo her principles, emphasizing the importance of combating inflammation, a key factor in many health issues, through natural, nourishing ingredients.

By scanning this QR code, you will unlock a series of engaging and informative videos. Each one is designed to provide you with step-by-step instructions on preparing anti-inflammatory meals and remedies. These recipes are not just beneficial for your health; they are also a delight to prepare and enjoy, bringing the essence of Barbara's teachings into your kitchen and daily life.

This bonus is an extension of the book's mission to empower you with knowledge and skills for a healthier life. It offers a hands-on experience, allowing you to apply the teachings of Dr. O'Neill in practical, tangible ways. Whether you are a beginner in the kitchen or an experienced cook, these video recipes will add a new dimension to your understanding of anti-inflammatory foods and how to incorporate them into your diet.

We invite you to scan this QR code and immerse yourself in the world of natural, health-boosting cuisine. Let these video recipes inspire you, enhance your culinary skills, and bring the essence of Barbara's holistic health approach into your everyday life.

Embark on this culinary journey with an open heart and a curious palate, and discover the power of food in promoting health and well-being, just as Barbara O'Neill has always advocated.

@ANTIINFLAMMATORYDIET.OFFICIAL

Chapter 3: Detoxification

Barbara O'Neill's perspective on detoxification is deeply rooted in a holistic and natural approach to health and well-being. She firmly believes in the body's remarkable ability to detoxify itself through its inherent systems and processes. In her view, the key to effective detoxification lies in providing the body with the optimal conditions to support and enhance its innate cleansing mechanisms.

Central to O'Neill's philosophy is the recognition that the human body possesses its own detoxification systems, primarily involving organs such as the liver, kidneys, skin, and the gastrointestinal tract. These vital organs work synergistically to process and eliminate toxins and waste products from the body. O'Neill emphasizes the importance of nurturing and strengthening these natural detox pathways through a combination of lifestyle choices, dietary habits, and mindful practices.

Her approach to detoxification places a significant emphasis on the role of nutrition. O'Neill advocates for a diet that is grounded in whole, natural foods, particularly plant-based choices that are rich in essential nutrients and antioxidants. She believes that such a diet not only provides the body with the necessary nutrients for optimal functioning but also supports its natural detox mechanisms.

Hydration is another critical aspect of O'Neill's detoxification philosophy. She underscores the importance of maintaining adequate hydration to facilitate the efficient removal of toxins from the body. Clean, filtered water is regarded as an essential component of the detoxification process.

Stress management is a fundamental part of O'Neill's approach to holistic health and detoxification. She recognizes the adverse effects of chronic stress on the body's ability to detoxify and encourages practices such as deep breathing, meditation, and relaxation techniques as valuable tools in maintaining overall well-being.

In summary, Barbara O'Neill's perspective on detoxification revolves around empowering the body to harness its own natural detoxifying abilities. Her philosophy is grounded in the belief that by adopting a balanced, whole-foods-based diet, staying hydrated, managing stress, and cultivating a holistic lifestyle, individuals can create an environment in which the body can thrive and efficiently rid itself of toxins. Her teachings emphasize the profound connection between a natural, healthy lifestyle and the body's innate capacity for detoxification and self-healing.

Delving into the science of detoxification, we uncover a world where our bodies function with remarkable precision and complexity to maintain health and equilibrium. This sophisticated system, often simplified in popular wellness culture, is a symphony of biological processes, each orchestrated to ensure that toxins, both external and internal, are effectively neutralized and eliminated…but, who are the players in this detoxification challenge? Let's know them better!

Liver: The Biochemical Transformer

The liver, often referred to as the body's biochemical transformer, is an organ of monumental importance in the detoxification process, performing a series of complex and multifaceted functions that are crucial for maintaining health. To delve deeper into its role is to uncover a world of intricate biochemical processes that underscore the sophistication of human physiology.

Phase I of liver detoxification, primarily involving the cytochrome P450 enzyme family, is a fascinating showcase of biochemical ingenuity. These enzymes, acting as catalysts, embark on the process of biotransformation, wherein they modify the chemical structure of toxins, preparing them for further processing. It's a process akin to preparing a rough diamond for the final cut and polish. The enzymes introduce a reactive group into the toxin, which often results in the formation of a free radical – a highly reactive molecule.

This creation of free radicals is a double-edged sword; while it's a necessary step in rendering toxins more water-soluble, it also poses a risk of cellular damage. Herein lies the critical role of antioxidants, substances that neutralize free radicals. The body's natural antioxidants, like glutathione, along with dietary antioxidants from fruits and vegetables, come into play, safeguarding the body's cells from potential oxidative damage. This delicate balance maintained in the liver highlights the organ's intricate response system and underscores the importance of a nutrient-rich diet to support these processes.

Following Phase I, the liver initiates Phase II detoxification, a phase that is less about modification and more about conjugation. In this phase, the liver cells attach various substances to the toxin, further increasing its water solubility. This conjugation reaction involves pathways such as glucuronidation, sulfation, and methylation, each utilizing different molecules to neutralize toxins.

Glucuronidation attaches glucuronic acid to toxins, making them more water-soluble. Sulfation, as the name suggests, involves the addition of sulfate groups. Methylation, another crucial pathway, uses methyl groups to further process the toxins. The efficiency of these pathways is dependent on the availability of certain nutrients in the body, such as sulfur-containing amino acids for sulfation and B-vitamins for methylation. This reliance on nutrients is a vivid reminder of how our diet directly influences the body's capacity to detoxify.

The health of the liver is vital for overall well-being. Factors such as poor diet, excessive alcohol consumption, and exposure to environmental toxins can impair liver function, leading to a decreased ability to detoxify. This underscores the importance of lifestyle choices in maintaining liver health. Practices such as consuming a balanced diet rich in fruits, vegetables, and whole grains, staying hydrated, limiting alcohol intake, and reducing exposure to environmental toxins are pivotal in supporting liver function.

In the broader context of holistic health, the liver's role as a biochemical transformer is a prime example of the body's natural resilience and intelligence. It's a complex system, finely tuned and capable of remarkable feats of biochemistry, essential for life. Understanding and supporting this system through our dietary and lifestyle choices is a testament to the interconnectedness of our bodies and the environments in which we live. The liver, in its silent yet crucial role, not only protects us from toxins but also serves as a constant reminder of the body's incredible capacity for self-maintenance and healing.

Kidneys: The Filtration Maestros

The kidneys, often unsung heroes in the body's detoxification narrative, are masterful in their role as filtration maestros. These bean-shaped organs, each about the size of a fist, perform the critical function of filtering and purifying the blood, thus playing a pivotal role in the body's detoxification and waste elimination processes. To fully appreciate their function is to delve into a world of remarkable physiological processes and intricate systems that tirelessly work to maintain the body's delicate balance of fluids and electrolytes, and to remove waste products and toxins.

Every day, these powerful organs filter around 120 to 150 quarts of blood to produce about 1 to 2 quarts of urine. This urine contains waste products and toxins that the body needs to expel. The kidneys achieve this through a complex system of filtration units known as nephrons. Each kidney contains about a million nephrons, and each nephron is a microscopic world unto itself, consisting of a glomerulus and a tubule. The glomerulus is a network of tiny blood vessels where blood filtration begins. It acts like a sieve, keeping large molecules such as proteins and blood cells in the bloodstream while allowing smaller molecules, waste products, and excess fluids to pass through.

The role of the kidneys extends beyond filtration. They are also crucial in regulating the body's electrolyte levels, including sodium, potassium, and phosphate, which are vital for many bodily functions. They maintain the pH balance of the blood, ensuring it remains slightly alkaline, which is essential for optimal cellular function. This balancing act is a testament to the kidneys' precision and efficiency in maintaining homeostasis.

Moreover, the kidneys have a hormonal function. They produce erythropoietin, a hormone that stimulates the production of red blood cells, and renin, which regulates blood pressure. The kidneys' ability to control blood pressure is not only through the production of renin but also through the regulation of the volume of blood plasma, further illustrating their multifaceted role in the body's overall health.

Given their critical functions, maintaining kidney health is paramount. Factors such as chronic high blood pressure, diabetes, and exposure to certain toxins can impair kidney function. This leads to a reduced ability to filter blood effectively, resulting in the accumulation of waste products and imbalances in electrolytes and fluids, which can have widespread effects on the body.

To support kidney health, it's essential to consider dietary and lifestyle factors. Adequate hydration is crucial as it aids the kidneys in flushing out waste products. A diet that is low in sodium helps in maintaining healthy blood pressure, reducing the strain on the kidneys. Additionally, moderating protein intake can help decrease the workload on the kidneys, particularly in individuals with compromised kidney function.

In the context of holistic health, the role of the kidneys is a prime example of the body's intricate and interdependent systems. Their ability to filter blood, regulate vital substances, and maintain overall balance is integral to our health. Understanding and supporting these processes through mindful dietary and lifestyle choices is a reflection of a holistic approach to health, recognizing the kidneys not just as standalone organs but as integral components of a larger, interconnected system.

In conclusion, the kidneys, as the body's filtration maestros, perform their roles with remarkable precision and efficiency. Their contribution to detoxification, fluid and electrolyte balance, and overall bodily function is a marvel of human physiology. Caring for these vital organs through healthy lifestyle choices is not just a matter of kidney health but is essential for the well-being of the entire body. As we continue to explore the wonders of the human body, the kidneys stand as a testament to the complexity and resilience inherent in our biological systems.

Gastrointestinal System: The Unsung Hero

As someone who has delved into the depths of holistic health and the wonders of herbalism, I've come to recognize the gastrointestinal system's pivotal role in detoxification, a role that is as complex as it is vital.

The gastrointestinal system's role in detoxification begins with its function as the body's first line of defense against ingested toxins. The stomach, with its acidic environment, plays a key role in breaking down food and killing potential pathogens. As food travels through the digestive system, various enzymes and digestive juices further break it down, allowing the absorption of nutrients while simultaneously isolating and preparing toxins for elimination.

One of the most fascinating aspects of the GI tract's role in detoxification is the gut microbiome. This complex ecosystem, comprising billions of bacteria, is not only crucial for digesting certain types of fiber but also plays a role in metabolizing various substances that the body deems toxic. These beneficial bacteria can transform toxins into less harmful substances, which can then be safely excreted. Furthermore, a healthy gut microbiome is essential for maintaining the integrity of the gut lining, preventing the leakage of harmful substances into the bloodstream.

The detoxification process within the gastrointestinal system is intricately linked with liver function, a connection often referred to as the liver-gut axis. Substances absorbed from the gut are first transported to the liver, where they undergo further detoxification. This relationship highlights the importance of maintaining both liver and gut health for effective detoxification.

However, the GI system's ability to perform these functions can be compromised by factors such as poor diet, chronic stress, and the use of certain medications. These factors can disrupt the gut microbiome, impair digestive functions, and lead to conditions such as leaky gut syndrome, where toxins and partially digested food particles escape into the bloodstream, increasing the body's toxic burden.

Supporting gastrointestinal health is thus a cornerstone of effective detoxification. This includes consuming a diet rich in fiber, which not only aids in the movement of food through the digestive tract but also supports the health of the gut microbiome. Hydration is crucial, as water helps in the digestive process and the efficient elimination of waste. Probiotic-rich foods and prebiotics are also vital, as they support the growth and health of beneficial gut bacteria.

In herbalism, various plants are recognized for their benefits to the gastrointestinal system. Herbs like ginger and peppermint can aid digestion, while others like slippery elm and marshmallow root can help in maintaining the integrity of the gut lining. These herbs, used thoughtfully, can be powerful allies in supporting gastrointestinal health.

In conclusion, the gastrointestinal system's role in detoxification is multifaceted and indispensable. Its health is fundamental not just for efficient detoxification but for the overall well-being of the body. Understanding and supporting this complex system through diet, lifestyle, and natural remedies is a testament to the holistic approach to health, recognizing the interconnectedness of our body's systems and the importance of nurturing each part to support the whole; the gastrointestinal system remains a crucial area of focus, a true unsung hero in our journey towards health and vitality.

Skin and Lungs: Peripheral Detox Players

Their roles exemplify the body's comprehensive approach to maintaining purity and balance, showcasing the sophisticated interplay of various systems working in harmony to expel toxins.

The skin, the body's largest organ, is a dynamic barrier protecting against external toxins and microorganisms. Beyond this protective function, it plays a significant role in the detoxification process through perspiration. Sweating, more than a cooling mechanism, is a route for the elimination of waste products including salts, urea, and, in some cases, heavy metals like lead and mercury. The act of sweating not only helps to regulate body temperature but also serves to rid the body of certain toxins, aiding in overall detoxification.

The health of the skin is crucial in ensuring its effectiveness as a detox organ. Factors such as hydration, nutrition, and skin hygiene all play vital roles. Staying adequately hydrated ensures that the sweat glands function optimally, while a diet rich in essential nutrients helps maintain the skin's health and resilience. Herbal remedies, known for their skin-beneficial properties, like chamomile and calendula, can be used in skincare to support the skin's detoxifying functions.

The lungs, primarily associated with the vital function of oxygenating the blood, also play a crucial role in detoxification. Every breath inhaled not only brings in oxygen but also exposes the body to airborne pollutants and particles. The lungs act as guardians, filtering out harmful particles through a lining of mucus and a system of fine hairs, or cilia, which trap and help expel these particles from the respiratory tract.

One of the most remarkable aspects of lung function is the exchange of gases that occurs within the alveoli, tiny air sacs in the lungs. Here, carbon dioxide, a waste product of metabolism, is exchanged for oxygen. This process is fundamental to life and highlights the lungs' role in maintaining the body's biochemical balance.

Environmental factors, such as air quality, and lifestyle choices, like smoking, significantly impact lung health and, consequently, their ability to function effectively in detoxification. Practices such as deep breathing exercises, regular physical activity, and exposure to clean, fresh air are beneficial in supporting lung health. Additionally, certain herbs known for their respiratory benefits, such as eucalyptus and peppermint, can be used to support lung function.

In the broader context of detoxification, supporting the health of the skin and lungs is as crucial as supporting the liver or kidneys. This involves not only direct care through skincare and respiratory health practices but also an overall lifestyle that minimizes exposure to toxins. For the skin, this might mean using natural skincare products and protecting it from excessive sun exposure. For the lungs, it might involve creating a living environment with clean air, free from pollutants and allergens, and avoiding smoking.

In conclusion, the roles of the skin and lungs in the body's detoxification process are significant and multifaceted. They highlight the body's remarkable capacity to adapt and cleanse itself through various mechanisms. Understanding and supporting these organs through holistic health practices, dietary choices, and lifestyle modifications are key components of a comprehensive approach to detoxification and overall well-being. As we continue to explore and appreciate the body's complex detoxification systems, the skin and lungs stand as vital players, each contributing uniquely to the maintenance of health and balance within the body.

The Lymphatic System

At the heart of Dr. O'Neill's discussion is the lymphatic system, a critical but often overlooked component of our body's wellness. She likens the lymphatic system to a vacuum cleaner, emphasizing its role in sweeping out waste from the tissues and transporting it to the lymph nodes for disposal. This system, comprised of a network of vessels and nodes, is integral to maintaining internal cleanliness and balance. It works tirelessly to remove toxins and waste products from the cellular environment, playing a vital role in the body's defense mechanism.

Blood plays a paramount role in maintaining the health and vitality of our bodies, a fact that Dr. O'Neill stresses in her teachings. It is the vehicle that carries essential oxygen and nutrients to every cell, facilitating their proper function and ensuring their survival. The importance of blood in healing cannot be overstated; it is the medium through which the components necessary for repair and regeneration are delivered to various parts of the body. Rich in oxygen and nutrients, blood is the lifeline that sustains the intricate cellular processes that underpin our health.

Within our blood resides our internal army – the immune system. Dr. O'Neill highlights the significance of the immune system, housed within our blood, as a key player in health and healing. This system is composed of various cells and proteins, always on the alert to identify and eliminate harmful pathogens that pose a threat to our well-being. It is a sophisticated defense mechanism, capable of mounting responses to a myriad of foreign invaders, thus safeguarding our bodies from infections and diseases.

In her teachings, Dr. O'Neill advocates for the use of natural substances to support the blood and lymphatic systems. She emphasizes the benefits of green barley, spirulina, and wheatgrass, particularly highlighting their high chlorophyll content. Chlorophyll, known for its great cleansing action, is effective in purifying the blood and tissues. These natural cleansers work by enhancing the elimination of toxins and supporting the body's natural detoxification processes. The inclusion of these superfoods in one's diet can significantly bolster the body's ability to maintain purity and equilibrium in the bloodstream and tissues.

An intriguing aspect of Dr. O'Neill's recommendations is the practice of rebounding, particularly in the morning, to activate the lymphatic system. Rebounding, which involves bouncing on a mini-trampoline, is an effective way to stimulate the lymphatic system. This gentle yet dynamic exercise causes the valves in the lymphatic system to open and close simultaneously, enhancing lymph flow and aiding in the removal of toxins. By incorporating rebounding into a daily routine, one can significantly improve the efficiency of the body's 'vacuum cleaner', ensuring the timely and effective removal of waste from the tissues.

In conclusion, Dr. Barbara O'Neill's insights into the blood and lymphatic systems reveal the profound wisdom of our bodies' natural processes. Her teachings encourage us to adopt practices and diets that support these systems, thereby enhancing our overall health and well-being. Understanding the vital roles played by the lymphatic and blood systems is not just about recognizing their functions but also about appreciating the intricate balance and harmony within our bodies. By aligning our lifestyles with these natural processes, we can foster a deeper connection with our bodies, leading to a healthier, more vibrant existence.

Dr. O'Neill emphasizes the immune system's role as the body's primary defense against illness and infection. It operates like a well-coordinated army, sending lymphatic fluid, extra blood, and white blood cells to areas of injury or infection. This rapid mobilization is crucial in preventing the spread of harmful microbes and initiating the healing process. The lymphatic fluid serves as a transportation medium, while white blood cells, the soldiers of the immune system, are instrumental in combating invaders and protecting the body from potential threats.

The role of the nose in the immune system is often overlooked, yet Dr. O'Neill sheds light on its significance. The nose, with its little cavities and hairs, acts as a natural filtration system, effectively filtering out dust and particles from the air we breathe. This mechanism ensures that only clean, particle-free air reaches the lungs. Such filtering is crucial in preventing airborne pathogens and irritants from entering the respiratory tract, thereby playing a vital role in maintaining respiratory health.

A fascinating aspect of the immune system, as highlighted by Dr. O'Neill, is the role of hydrochloric acid in our stomach. This potent acid is not only essential for digestion but also serves as a formidable barrier against pathogens. By wiping out harmful bacteria and viruses that enter our body through ingested food or drink, hydrochloric acid is a key player in the immune defense, safeguarding our internal environment from potential infections.

At Misty Mountain Health Retreat, a unique practice involves diving into a cold creek, an experience that may elicit screams but is said to strongly stimulate the immune system. This sudden exposure to cold water is believed to trigger a shock response in the body, activating the immune system. Such stimulation can lead to an increased production of white blood cells and other components of the immune system, potentially enhancing its ability to fight off infections and diseases. This practice is an example of how environmental stressors, in controlled situations, can be used to bolster the body's natural defense mechanisms.

In summary, the immune system's functions and mechanisms are complex and multifaceted, playing a crucial role in maintaining our health and well-being. Dr. O'Neill's insights into the immune system illuminate the various natural defenses our bodies possess and highlight the importance of supporting these systems through our lifestyle choices. Understanding the immune system's workings is not just about recognizing its components and functions but also about appreciating the delicate balance it maintains in protecting us from the myriad of challenges it faces daily. By aligning our lifestyles with practices that support and enhance the immune system, we can foster greater health and resilience against illnesses.

Q&A

What exactly is the immune system, and what is its function?

— The immune system serves as the primary defense against harmful organisms, beginning with the skin, which acts as a protective shield. In response to infection or injury, it mobilizes white blood cells to the impacted areas for protection.

What are some ways to enhance my immune system naturally?

— Improving your immune system can be achieved through dietary habits, physical activity, and overall lifestyle modifications. Embracing a diet rich in plant-based foods, ensuring adequate hydration, and engaging in regular physical exercise can bolster immune health.

What natural methods exist for alleviating pain and inflammation?

— Alternating between hot and cold water treatments, followed by applying a potato poultice, can effectively reduce pain and inflammation, avoiding the side effects associated with medications. This approach promotes circulation and triggers the body's inherent healing mechanisms.

Does cutting out specific foods from my diet benefit my health?

— Removing gluten and dairy from your diet can potentially enhance memory, reduce symptoms such as brain fog and bloating, and contribute to overall health improvement. It's advisable to eliminate these food groups temporarily to assess any sensitivities.

What steps can I take to improve my water's quality?

— Enhancing your water's quality can be achieved by allowing chlorine to evaporate naturally by leaving water out, and employing filtration techniques like reverse osmosis or ceramic filters to eliminate harmful elements like fluoride. Consuming pure water plays a crucial role in sustaining robust immune health.

Dietary Approaches to Detoxification

When it comes to maintaining optimal health and well-being, few aspects of our lives are as crucial as our diet. What we eat plays a significant role in determining not only our physical health but also our mental and emotional well-being. It's no wonder that the adage "You are what you eat" holds true in countless ways.

Barbara O'Neill stands as a beacon of wisdom and guidance. Her teachings emphasize the importance of nurturing our bodies with wholesome, natural foods that support our innate cleansing and detoxification processes. Barbara O'Neill's approach to nutrition is rooted in the belief that the right foods can not only nourish us but also help cleanse and heal our bodies from the inside out.

This table is a comprehensive guide to some of the foods that Barbara O'Neill recommends for promoting cleansing and detoxification. It delves into various categories of foods, from fruits and vegetables to legumes, nuts, and herbs and spices. Each category contains specific examples of foods that possess unique properties to aid in detoxification and support overall health.

Let's explore these categories and the benefits of the foods they contain:

Fruits have long been celebrated for their nutritional value, and Barbara O'Neill highlights their role in supporting detoxification. Citrus fruits like lemons and oranges are rich in vitamin C, a powerful antioxidant known to support liver detoxification. Berries such as blueberries and strawberries provide antioxidants and fiber, aiding in the removal of toxins. Apples, with their natural pectin content, act as natural detoxifiers, supporting digestive health.

Barbara O'Neill encourages the consumption of a variety of vegetables, especially leafy greens like kale and spinach. These greens are abundant in chlorophyll, which supports liver and blood cleansing. Beets contain betalains, compounds that promote liver health, while carrots are rich in beta-carotene, a potent antioxidant. Cruciferous vegetables like broccoli and kale support liver enzymes involved in detoxification, and garlic and onions contain sulfur compounds that aid in detoxification.

Lentils, chickpeas, and beans (such as black and kidney beans) are excellent sources of both fiber and protein. They play a vital role in supporting colon cleansing and promoting digestive health. Barbara O'Neill recommends including these legumes and pulses in your diet to facilitate toxin removal.

Nuts and seeds offer a combination of healthy fats and detoxifying properties. Almonds, rich in vitamin E, support skin health and cleansing. Chia seeds are packed with fiber and omega-3 fatty acids, aiding digestion and overall well-being. Flaxseeds contain lignans, which contribute to digestive health, while sunflower seeds provide essential minerals and vitamin E, supporting the body's cleansing processes.

Barbara O'Neill recognizes the significance of herbs and spices in promoting detoxification. Turmeric, containing curcumin, serves as a potent anti-inflammatory and detoxifier. Ginger supports digestion and possesses anti-inflammatory properties. Cilantro acts as a natural chelator, helping remove heavy metals from the body, while dandelion supports liver and kidney function and acts as a diuretic.

Hydration is key to any detoxification process, and Barbara O'Neill recommends specific beverages to support overall health and detoxification. Green tea, rich in antioxidants, promotes metabolism and detoxification. Herbal teas, such as dandelion and nettle, contribute to liver and kidney health, aiding in detoxification. Lemon water alkalizes the body, supports digestion, and enhances cleansing. Aloe vera juice soothes the digestive tract and promotes detoxification.

This table serves as a valuable resource for those seeking to embrace a diet that aligns with Barbara O'Neill's teachings on natural health and wholesome living. It's a testament to the notion that our choices in food can profoundly impact our body's ability to cleanse, rejuvenate, and thrive.

As you explore the foods in this table, remember that individual responses to foods may vary. It's essential to consult with a healthcare professional before making significant dietary changes, especially if you have underlying health conditions or allergies. Barbara O'Neill's guidance provides a foundation for understanding the power of cleansing foods, but personalized health decisions should always be made with care and consideration.

With this table as your reference, embark on a journey towards better health, one nourishing bite at a time. Let Barbara O'Neill's wisdom and the cleansing properties of these foods guide you on a path to holistic well-being.

Category	Food Examples	Benefits
Fruits	Citrus fruits (lemons, oranges)	Rich in vitamin C, supports liver detoxification
Fruits	Berries (blueberries, strawberries)	High in antioxidants and fiber, aid in toxin removal
Fruits	Apples	Contains pectin, a natural detoxifier
Vegetables	Leafy greens (kale, spinach)	Abundant in chlorophyll, supports liver and blood cleansing
Vegetables	Beets	Contains betalains, which support liver health
Vegetables	Carrots	Rich in beta-carotene, a powerful antioxidant
Vegetables	Cruciferous vegetables (broccoli, kale)	Support liver enzymes for detoxification
Vegetables	Garlic and onions	Contain sulfur compounds that aid detoxification
Legumes and Pulses	Lentils	High in fiber and protein, support colon cleansing
Legumes and Pulses	Chickpeas	Rich in fiber and protein, promote digestive health
Legumes and Pulses	Beans (black, kidney)	Provide protein and fiber, support toxin removal
Nuts and Seeds	Almonds	High in vitamin E and healthy fats, support skin cleansing
Nuts and Seeds	Chia seeds	Rich in fiber and omega-3 fatty acids, aid digestion

Nuts and Seeds	Flaxseeds	Contain lignans, support digestive health
Nuts and Seeds	Sunflower seeds	Provide vitamin E and essential minerals, aid in cleansing
Herbs and Spices	Turmeric	Contains curcumin, a potent anti-inflammatory and detoxifier
Herbs and Spices	Ginger	Supports digestion and has anti-inflammatory properties
Herbs and Spices	Cilantro	Acts as a natural chelator, helping remove heavy metals
Herbs and Spices	Dandelion	Supports liver and kidney function, acts as a diuretic
Beverages	Green tea	Rich in antioxidants, supports metabolism and detoxification
Beverages	Herbal teas (e.g., dandelion, nettle)	Promote liver and kidney health, aid in detoxification
Beverages	Lemon water	Alkalizes the body, supports digestion and cleansing
Beverages	Aloe vera juice	Soothes the digestive tract and promotes detoxification

Balancing Detox with Nutritional Needs

Nutritional needs refer to the specific dietary requirements that an individual's body requires to function optimally and maintain good health. These needs encompass the essential nutrients, vitamins, minerals, and energy (calories) that the body needs to perform various physiological functions, support growth and development, and prevent nutritional deficiencies and health problems.

Key components of nutritional needs include:

Macronutrients: These are the major nutrients that the body requires in relatively large amounts:

- Carbohydrates: Provide energy.

- Proteins: Essential for tissue repair, immune function, and enzyme production.

- Fats: Important for energy storage, cell structure, and the absorption of fat-soluble vitamins.

Micronutrients: These are vitamins and minerals that the body needs in smaller quantities but are crucial for various physiological processes:

- Vitamins (e.g., vitamin C, vitamin D, vitamin B-complex): Support functions like immune response, bone health, and energy metabolism.

- Minerals (e.g., calcium, iron, potassium): Play roles in bone health, oxygen transport, and electrolyte balance.

Water: Adequate hydration is essential for overall health and is considered a vital nutrient. It supports various bodily functions, including digestion, temperature regulation, and the transport of nutrients and waste products.

Caloric Intake: The body requires a certain number of calories (energy) to maintain its basic functions and activities. The caloric intake should align with an individual's age, sex, activity level, and overall health goals.

Fiber: Dietary fiber is essential for digestive health, regular bowel movements, and the prevention of conditions like constipation and diverticulitis.

Essential Fatty Acids: Certain fats, such as omega-3 and omega-6 fatty acids, are considered essential because the body cannot produce them on its own. They play roles in brain function, heart health, and inflammation regulation.

Antioxidants: These are compounds found in foods like fruits and vegetables that help protect the body from oxidative stress and free radicals, which can contribute to chronic diseases.

Meeting nutritional needs is crucial for overall well-being, as it ensures that the body receives the necessary nutrients to maintain proper growth, repair tissues, support the immune system, and prevent nutritional deficiencies or health issues. The specific nutritional needs of an individual can vary based on factors such as age, gender, activity level, underlying health conditions, and dietary preferences. As a result, it's important to have a balanced and varied diet that provides all the essential nutrients required for optimal health.

Barbara O'Neill's teachings emphasize not only the importance of detoxification but also the crucial need to balance it with our nutritional requirements. While detoxifying the body is a vital aspect of maintaining good health, it should be approached with mindfulness to ensure that our bodies receive the essential nutrients they need for optimal functioning.

Barbara O'Neill acknowledges that our modern lifestyles expose us to various toxins and pollutants, ranging from environmental contaminants to processed foods. These toxins can accumulate in our bodies over time and compromise our health. Hence, she advocates for detoxification as a means to rid the body of these harmful substances.

However, Barbara O'Neill's approach to detoxification is far from extreme or deprivation-based. She believes in a balanced approach that combines the removal of toxins with the provision of vital nutrients. Here are some key principles and insights from her perspective:

Whole Foods as the Foundation: Barbara O'Neill's teachings consistently underscore the importance of whole foods in our diet. These foods are not only nutritious but also supportive of the body's natural detoxification processes. Fruits, vegetables, legumes, nuts, and seeds are rich in vitamins, minerals, and antioxidants that nourish our bodies while aiding in detoxification.

Variety and Balance: Barbara O'Neill encourages a diverse and balanced diet that includes a wide range of natural, plant-based foods. This diversity ensures that we receive a spectrum of nutrients while supporting various detoxification pathways in the body.

Hydration for Detox: Adequate hydration is a cornerstone of detoxification. Barbara O'Neill recommends beverages such as green tea, herbal teas, and lemon water as they not only help flush out toxins but also provide hydration, essential for overall well-being.

Mindful Detox: Rather than endorsing extreme detox diets or fasting, Barbara O'Neill emphasizes the importance of mindful detox. This involves making conscious choices to minimize exposure to toxins and adopting a diet rich in foods that naturally support detoxification.

Nutrient-Rich Superfoods: While advocating for a balanced diet, Barbara O'Neill also recognizes the value of nutrient-dense superfoods. These foods, such as turmeric, ginger, and leafy greens, are known for their exceptional health benefits and detoxifying properties.

Supplementation with Caution: While Barbara O'Neill believes in the power of natural supplements and herbal remedies, she advises caution when using supplements. It's important not to rely solely on supplements for detoxification but rather incorporate them as part of a well-rounded diet.

Consulting Healthcare Professionals: Barbara O'Neill emphasizes the importance of consulting healthcare professionals, particularly if one has specific health conditions or dietary restrictions. Balancing detox with nutritional needs should be tailored to individual circumstances.

Long-Term Lifestyle Change: Barbara O'Neill's teachings promote long-term lifestyle changes rather than quick fixes. She encourages individuals to adopt sustainable dietary habits that align with their health goals and support ongoing detoxification.

In conclusion, Barbara O'Neill's perspective on balancing detox with nutritional needs is rooted in the idea that the body has a remarkable capacity to cleanse and heal itself when provided with the right tools. Her teachings promote a holistic approach to health, where detoxification is seamlessly integrated into a nourishing and sustainable dietary lifestyle. By embracing the wisdom shared by Barbara O'Neill, individuals can embark on a exploration towards improved health and well-being while respecting the body's inherent need for both detox and nourishment.

Example	Ingredients and Instructions
Green Smoothie Detox	- Leafy greens (e.g., spinach, kale, chard) - Detox herbs (e.g., cilantro, parsley) - Fruits (e.g., berries, banana) - Blend ingredients for a nutrient-packed breakfast.
Turmeric and Ginger Elixir	- Turmeric and ginger - Warm water - Make a soothing tea to support liver function and reduce inflammation.
Fiber-Rich Salad	- Leafy greens - Carrots - Beets - Chickpeas or black beans - Lemon juice and olive oil dressing - Combine for a fiber-rich salad that balances detox and nutrition.
Hydration and Lemon Water	- Warm water - Lemon juice - Start your day with a glass to alkalize the body and provide vitamin C.
Detoxifying Herbs in Cooking	- Cilantro, ginger, etc. - Use herbs and spices in everyday cooking for added flavor and detox support.
Balanced Detox Smoothie	- Kale, cucumber, dandelion greens - Almond butter - Flaxseeds - Blend for a balanced detox and nutritional smoothie.
Detoxifying Soup	- Vegetable-based soup with garlic, onions, and colorful vegetables - Lentils or chickpeas - Make a hearty, detoxifying soup.
Mindful Food Choices	- Avoid processed foods, artificial additives, and excessive sugar - Choose natural, whole foods for daily detox support.

Detoxification through Fasting

Fasting initiates a fascinating series of transformations within our body, and these changes are rooted in the body's remarkable ability to adapt and maintain balance, which aligns with Barbara O'Neill's holistic philosophy.

To begin, when we cease food intake during a fast, our body experiences a decrease in insulin levels. This is because insulin is primarily released in response to food consumption to regulate glucose levels. With lowered insulin, the body transitions to a state where it can tap into its internal energy reserves.

The first energy store to be utilized is glycogen, stored in the liver and muscles. As we fast, these glycogen stores are gradually depleted to provide a steady supply of glucose to sustain essential bodily functions and maintain blood sugar levels.

As glycogen reserves are utilized, the body enters a state known as ketosis. This is a pivotal phase where the liver starts breaking down fats into ketone molecules, which serve as an alternative energy source, especially for the brain. It's a fascinating metabolic shift that supports energy production while fasting.

Another intriguing aspect of fasting is the process of autophagy. Fasting triggers autophagy, a cellular recycling mechanism. During autophagy, the body identifies and removes damaged or dysfunctional cellular components, contributing to overall cellular health and rejuvenation. This aligns with Barbara O'Neill's holistic emphasis on the body's innate capacity for self-healing.

Furthermore, fasting encourages the body to turn to stored fat for energy. This gradual fat utilization can lead to fat loss, making fasting a popular approach for those seeking weight management.

Hormonal changes also come into play during fasting. Human growth hormone (HGH), known for its roles in muscle preservation and fat burning, increases in response to fasting. Additionally, norepinephrine levels rise, further promoting the breakdown of fats.

Beyond these metabolic shifts, fasting allows the body to channel its resources toward cellular repair and regeneration. This includes DNA repair, cellular membrane maintenance, and the restoration of vital cellular components, promoting holistic well-being.

Intriguingly, some studies suggest that fasting may contribute to the reduction of inflammation in the body, which is associated with various chronic health concerns. This aligns with Barbara O'Neill's holistic approach, which aims to address the root causes of health issues.

Finally, fasting can enhance insulin sensitivity, making it easier for cells to respond to insulin and regulate blood sugar levels. This improvement in insulin sensitivity can reduce the risk of insulin resistance and type 2 diabetes.

Fasting is a multifaceted process that engages the body's natural mechanisms for energy utilization, cellular repair, and overall well-being. Barbara O'Neill's holistic philosophy underscores the body's ability to self-regulate and heal, and fasting can be seen as a way to support these innate processes when approached mindfully and in alignment with individual health goals. However, it's crucial to remember that fasting may not be suitable for everyone, and consulting with a healthcare provider who shares holistic principles akin to Barbara O'Neill's is advisable before embarking on a fasting experience.

Barbara O'Neill, a prominent advocate for natural health and holistic living, approaches fasting in a manner that aligns with her holistic principles. Although specific quotes or writings from her are not available to me, I can offer insights based on her holistic teachings.

In Barbara O'Neill's holistic framework, fasting can be seen as a natural and time-tested practice. It's regarded as a method through which the body engages in self-purification and detoxification. By abstaining from food for a defined period, the digestive system is allowed to rest, and the body can redirect its energy toward healing and regeneration.

Moreover, fasting is likely viewed by Barbara O'Neill as a way to support the body's inherent capacity for self-healing. It enables the body to focus its resources on repairing tissues, eliminating accumulated toxins, and revitalizing cells. This perspective emphasizes the body's remarkable ability to restore balance and health when provided with the opportunity.

Barbara O'Neill's holistic approach to fasting likely underscores the importance of maintaining a balance between fasting and nutrition. While fasting can offer benefits, it should be approached in a well-planned manner that ensures essential nutrients are still provided when necessary. This approach ensures that fasting contributes to overall health and vitality.

Furthermore, mindfulness and intuition are central to holistic health. Barbara O'Neill may suggest that individuals should approach fasting mindfully, being attuned to their bodies and recognizing when fasting is appropriate. This aligns with the holistic philosophy of listening to one's body and responding to its unique needs.

Importantly, Barbara O'Neill's approach to fasting emphasizes that it should not be a one-size-fits-all practice. Each individual's body is distinct, and fasting should be personalized based on factors such as age, health status, and lifestyle. Tailoring fasting practices to individual circumstances is in line with her holistic philosophy.

Lastly, Barbara O'Neill's teachings frequently emphasize the significance of whole, natural foods. It is likely that she recommends breaking a fast with nutrient-rich, whole foods to ensure the body receives essential nourishment and supports the holistic approach to well-being.

It's essential to recognize that Barbara O'Neill's specific viewpoints on fasting can be found in her writings, lectures, or teachings. Her holistic philosophy focuses on natural health, nutrition, and lifestyle choices that promote overall well-being. Before engaging in any fasting regimen, it is advisable to seek guidance from a qualified healthcare provider or practitioner who aligns with the principles of Barbara O'Neill.

What is intermittent fasting, and how does it work?

Intermittent fasting is a dietary approach that has gained popularity in recent years and is often discussed within the world of natural health and holistic living, inspired by teachings like those of Barbara O'Neill. It involves cycling between periods of eating and fasting, with the primary focus on when you eat rather than what you eat.

The fundamental idea behind intermittent fasting is to create specific windows of time for eating and fasting. During the fasting periods, the body goes without calorie intake for an extended period, allowing it to tap into stored energy reserves for fuel. This process encourages various physiological changes:

Insulin Sensitivity: Fasting can improve insulin sensitivity, which means the body can use glucose more effectively, potentially reducing the risk of type 2 diabetes.

Cellular Repair: Fasting triggers a cellular repair process known as autophagy. During this process, the body removes damaged cells and regenerates new ones, contributing to overall cellular health.

Hormone Regulation: Intermittent fasting may affect hormone levels, including human growth hormone (HGH) and norepinephrine, which play roles in fat burning and metabolism.

Weight Management: By limiting the eating window, intermittent fasting can naturally reduce calorie intake, which may lead to weight loss or weight maintenance.

Inflammation Reduction: Some studies suggest that intermittent fasting can help reduce inflammation in the body, which is associated with various chronic diseases.

There are several popular methods of intermittent fasting, such as the 16/8 method (fasting for 16 hours and eating during an 8-hour window), the 5:2 diet (eating normally for five days and consuming very few calories on two non-consecutive days), and alternate-day fasting (alternating between fasting days and regular eating days).

It's important to note that intermittent fasting may not be suitable for everyone, and individual experiences can vary. Factors like age, health status, and personal preferences should be considered when exploring this approach. Consulting with a healthcare provider or practitioner with knowledge of natural health practices, like those inspired by Barbara O'Neill, is advisable before starting any fasting regimen.

Different types of intermittent fasting

Intermittent fasting has gained recognition as a flexible dietary approach, and it aligns with Barbara O'Neill's holistic philosophy, which emphasizes mindful and natural ways to support health.

The 16/8 Method: This is one of the most common forms of intermittent fasting. It involves fasting for 16 hours each day and restricting your eating to an 8-hour window. For example, you might eat between 12 PM and 8 PM and fast from 8 PM to 12 PM the following day.

The 5:2 Diet: In this approach, you consume your regular diet for five days of the week and significantly reduce calorie intake (usually around 500-600 calories) on two non-consecutive days. This method is flexible, allowing you to choose which days to fast.

Alternate-Day Fasting: As the name suggests, this schedule involves alternating between fasting days and regular eating days. On fasting days, calorie intake is minimal or nonexistent, while on eating days, you consume your usual meals.

The Eat-Stop-Eat Method: This method involves fasting for a full 24 hours once or twice a week. For example, you might fast from dinner one day to dinner the next day. It's important to stay hydrated during these fasts.

The Warrior Diet: This approach involves fasting for most of the day and having a small eating window in the evening. You might fast for 20 hours and eat during a 4-hour window in the evening.

The OMAD (One Meal A Day) Diet: With this method, you consume all your daily calories in one large meal, typically within a 1-2 hour window. The rest of the day is spent in fasting.

The 12/12 Method: This is one of the simplest forms of intermittent fasting. It involves a 12-hour fasting period followed by a 12-hour eating window. Many people choose to fast overnight, making it an easy schedule to adopt.

The 24-Hour Fast: Similar to the Eat-Stop-Eat method, this approach entails fasting for a full 24 hours once or twice a week. It offers flexibility in choosing which days to fast and is often combined with fasting from dinner to dinner.

The Extended Fasting: Some individuals embark on longer fasting periods, such as 36 hours or more. Extended fasting should be approached cautiously and may require medical supervision.

Each of these intermittent fasting schedules has its unique approach and potential benefits. The choice of which method to adopt should align with individual health goals, lifestyle, and preferences. It's essential to approach intermittent fasting mindfully, ensuring it complements your overall well-being and is carried out safely and in consultation with healthcare professionals who embrace holistic health principles similar to those advocated by Barbara O'Neill.

Is intermittent fasting safe for everyone?

Intermittent fasting is generally considered safe for many individuals and has been embraced by those seeking natural and holistic approaches to well-being. However, it's essential to recognize that not everyone is the same, and the suitability of intermittent fasting can vary based on individual circumstances.

Individual Variability: People have unique metabolic rates, nutritional needs, and health conditions. What works for one person may not be suitable for another. It's crucial to consider individual factors when deciding to adopt intermittent fasting.

Medical Conditions: Individuals with certain medical conditions, such as diabetes, eating disorders, or a history of heart issues, should exercise caution when considering intermittent fasting. Consultation with a healthcare provider who understands holistic health principles is advisable in such cases.

Medications: Some medications may require specific timing for intake with food. Fasting could interfere with the effectiveness of certain medications. Healthcare professionals can provide guidance on medication management during fasting.

Pregnancy and Nursing: Pregnant or nursing individuals have additional nutritional needs, and fasting may not be suitable during these times. It's essential to prioritize the health of both the mother and the child and seek guidance from healthcare providers experienced in holistic health approaches.

Age and Growth: Intermittent fasting may not be suitable for children and adolescents, as they are in stages of growth and development that require consistent nutrition.

Listen to Your Body: Regardless of individual circumstances, it's vital to listen to your body when practicing intermittent fasting. If fasting leads to excessive hunger, fatigue, dizziness, or other discomforts, it's essential to reevaluate the fasting approach.

Consult a Holistic Practitioner: For those who align with holistic health principles, consulting with a healthcare provider or holistic practitioner who understands these principles can be valuable. They can provide personalized guidance, considering not only the physical but also the mental and emotional aspects of well-being.

In essence, intermittent fasting can be a valuable tool for those seeking holistic approaches to health. However, it should always be approached mindfully, with an understanding of individual needs and a willingness to adapt the fasting schedule to ensure both safety and effectiveness. Ultimately, the key is to prioritize health and well-being, seeking guidance from healthcare professionals who share a holistic perspective, similar to the teachings of Barbara O'Neill.

Chapter 4: Herbal Remedies

The history of herbalism is intricately linked with the evolution of medicine, spanning from ancient times until the emergence of the germ theory of disease in the 19th century. It's a journey that reflects the development of human understanding and the harnessing of nature's remedies for healing.

In prehistoric eras, long before recorded history, humans were already tapping into the therapeutic potential of plants. The archaeological record provides fascinating insights into the use of medicinal plants during the Paleolithic period, approximately 60,000 years ago. Remarkably, this practice was not exclusive to humans; even non-human primates were observed using medicinal plants to address illnesses, demonstrating the deep-rooted connection between nature and healing.

Archaeological discoveries further bolster the idea that ancient peoples possessed knowledge of herbal medicine. For instance, a Neanderthal burial site called "Shanidar IV" in northern Iraq, dating back 60,000 years, yielded large amounts of pollen from eight plant species. Astonishingly, seven of these plants continue to be utilized today as herbal remedies, emphasizing the timelessness of herbal healing.

Fast forward to ancient civilizations, and we find the Sumerians in Mesopotamia, pioneers in the written study of herbs. Over 5,000 years ago, they inscribed clay tablets listing hundreds of medicinal plants, including myrrh and opium. These tablets provide evidence of an early systematization of herbal knowledge.

In the land of the pharaohs, ancient Egypt, herbalism merged with linguistic and translation complexities that have intrigued scholars for centuries. Texts like the Papyrus Ebers offer glimpses into ancient Egyptian herbal practices. This ancient manuscript lists over 850 plant medicines, including well-known herbs like garlic, juniper, and cannabis, along with lesser-known ones like castor bean and mandrake. Treatments were often directed at alleviating specific symptoms, as they were commonly perceived as the disease itself.

India, the cradle of Ayurveda, embraced herbal medicine over 1,000 years BCE. Early Sanskrit texts such as the Rig Veda and Atharva Veda laid the foundation for Ayurvedic herbalism. Visionaries like Charaka and Sushruta, during the 1st millennium BCE, documented their extensive knowledge of medicinal plants. The Sushruta Samhita alone describes 700 medicinal plants, 64 mineral-based preparations, and 57 sourced from animals.

In China, archaeological findings from the Bronze Age reveal seeds that likely played a role in herbalism. The legendary Chinese emperor Shennong authored the first Chinese pharmacopoeia, the "Shennong Ben Cao Jing," listing 365 medicinal plants, including the famous ephedra and hemp. Subsequent generations expanded on this compendium, exemplified by the Tang dynasty's "Yaoxing Lun."

Ancient Greece and Rome contributed significantly to herbalism. Hippocrates, often referred to as the 'Father of Western Medicine,' emphasized logic and reason in medical practices. The Hippocratic Corpus contains myriad herbal remedies, which differ from religious healing practices by their rational approach.

Galen of Pergamon, a Greek physician in Rome, left a profound impact with his extensive works on herbs. He delved into the concept of humors and the four basic qualities to better tailor treatments to individual needs.

Diocles of Carystus, sometimes dubbed "the second Hippocrates," added his insights to herbalism, but his original texts have been lost over time. Nevertheless, scholars have quoted him extensively.

Pliny the Elder's "Natural History" cataloged over 900 drugs and plants, providing an expansive knowledge base for herbalism. His writings reflected a holistic view of ailments and remedies within the context of nature's balance.

Pedanius Dioscorides created the influential "De Materia Medica," containing over 1,000 medicines derived from herbs, minerals, and animals. His work served as a cornerstone of herbal knowledge for over 1,600 years.

Herbalism thrived in the Middle Ages, despite debates among scholars about the intent and understanding behind medieval herbal documents. Some believed that medieval texts merely copied classical knowledge, while others argued for genuine understanding.

Benedictine monasteries were vital hubs of herbal knowledge in Europe. Notable figures like Hildegard of Bingen, a 12th-century Benedictine nun, contributed to herbal medicine with her work "Causae et Curae." Women played a significant role in herbalism, especially among Germanic tribes.

Overall, the history of herbalism reveals a profound and enduring connection between humanity and the healing power of nature. From prehistoric times to the Middle Ages, the knowledge of herbs and their applications evolved, leaving an indelible mark on the development of medicine.

Natural Healing Approaches and Remedies

One of the most striking aspects of her philosophy is the emphasis on harnessing the body's natural healing abilities, a theme that resonates through various aspects of her teachings.

Dr. O'Neill posits a fascinating theory about the body's response to temperature variations, particularly in the context of a steam sauna followed by immersion in a mountain stream. According to her, this practice can potentially spike the body's metabolic rate by an astonishing 400%. This remarkable increase is attributed to the body's physiological reaction to the drastic temperature change, activating various biological processes that boost metabolism. The concept is rooted in the understanding that our bodies are equipped with intricate mechanisms designed to adapt and respond to environmental stresses, such as temperature shifts. By alternating between hot and cold environments, we essentially stimulate these mechanisms, thereby enhancing metabolic functions.

In a similar vein, Dr. O'Neill discusses the therapeutic benefits of contrasting temperature treatments for pain relief. For instance, the simple act of plunging a finger into ice-cold water after exposure to hot water can reportedly reduce pain levels by up to 50% in just 12 minutes. This approach offers a natural alternative to pain management, free from the side effects often associated with conventional medication. The underlying principle here is that the sudden cold exposure helps to decrease inflammation and numb nerve endings, providing rapid pain relief.

Dr. O'Neill's approach to treatment consistently emphasizes empowering the body's innate healing abilities. This perspective is particularly evident in her stance on the use of antibiotics and painkillers. While not dismissing the importance of conventional medicine in certain scenarios, she advocates for a more balanced approach, where natural healing methods are given precedence. The idea is to support the body's natural defense systems rather than relying solely on pharmaceutical interventions.

An exemplary case of this philosophy is her recommendation for tackling common ailments like colds. Dr. O'Neill champions the use of natural herbs and ingredients, such as garlic, ginger, lemon, honey, eucalyptus oil, and cayenne pepper. These natural remedies, she asserts, can effectively combat a cold and even shorten its duration. The rationale behind this advice is that these ingredients possess inherent medicinal properties that can bolster the immune system and alleviate symptoms. For instance, garlic is known for its antimicrobial and antiviral qualities, while honey can soothe a sore throat. Eucalyptus oil serves as a decongestant, ginger aids in reducing inflammation, lemon provides a vitamin C boost, and cayenne pepper helps in clearing nasal congestion.

Furthermore, Dr. O'Neill suggests combining these ingredients to create what she terms a 'natural flu bomb' remedy. This potent concoction is designed to harness the synergistic effects of its components, providing a comprehensive defense against flu symptoms. In contrast to flu injections, which may contain mercury and are not guaranteed to prevent the flu, this natural remedy offers a holistic and chemical-free alternative.

Throughout her teachings, Dr. O'Neill consistently advocates for a return to nature and the wisdom it holds in healing and maintaining our health. Her approach is not just about treating symptoms but about understanding and harmonizing with the natural processes of our bodies. By adopting such practices, she suggests that we can achieve a state of health that is both sustainable and attuned to the natural rhythms of our bodies.

In summary, Dr. O'Neill's teachings offer a refreshing perspective on health and wellness. By exploring and embracing these natural methods, we are reminded of the incredible capacity of our bodies to heal and thrive, provided we create the right conditions and listen to the subtle cues they offer. Her insights encourage us to look beyond conventional medicine and discover the power and simplicity of natural healing, a journey that is not only about curing ailments but also about fostering a deep and enduring connection with our bodies and the natural world around us.

Barbara O'Neill, brings to the forefront a wealth of insights and wisdom that illuminate the profound connection between humanity and the healing power of nature. Her studies into the field of herbal medicine is a testament to the transformative potential of holistic wellness practices.

What makes Barbara's insights particularly intriguing is her deep reverence for the natural world. She paints a vivid picture of the lush landscapes where medicinal herbs thrive, and she teaches us to appreciate the intricate beauty of each plant. Take, for instance, her description of the vibrant purple echinacea blossoms swaying gracefully in the breeze or the fragrant lavender fields that evoke a sense of tranquility. These vivid descriptions inspire a profound respect for the botanical allies that offer their healing gifts to us.

Barbara's understanding of herbal medicine transcends mere knowledge; it is a profound respect for the ancient traditions that have long recognized the therapeutic potential of plants. She often delves into the rich tapestry of cultural practices from around the world, demonstrating how various societies have harnessed the healing properties of herbs for centuries. Her insights showcase the universality of herbal wisdom and its ability to transcend borders and time.

One of the most fascinating aspects of Barbara's work is her emphasis on the synergy of herbs. She doesn't view medicinal plants in isolation but rather as part of a harmonious ecosystem. Her insights into herbal combinations and formulations are akin to composing a symphony of healing. She illustrates how certain herbs complement each other, creating a powerful synergy that enhances their therapeutic effects. It's akin to the way different instruments in an orchestra harmonize to create a beautiful melody.

Barbara's insights also extend to the art of herbal preparation. She guides us through the intricate processes of crafting infusions, decoctions, tinctures, and extracts, revealing the alchemical transformation that occurs when herbs and liquids intertwine. Her teachings empower individuals to become herbal artisans, capable of creating their own healing elixirs.

Moreover, Barbara O'Neill's work is marked by a deep sense of responsibility toward the environment. She emphasizes sustainable and ethical harvesting practices, ensuring that the earth's precious botanical treasures are safeguarded for future generations. Her insights remind us of the delicate balance between human healing and environmental stewardship.

Barbara's insights are a beacon of light, illuminating the path toward holistic well-being. Her teachings resonate with those seeking a deeper connection with nature and a profound understanding of the healing potential that lies within the embrace of medicinal plants. Barbara O'Neill's legacy in the world of herbal medicine is a testament to the enduring wisdom of the natural world and its capacity to nurture and heal both body and soul.

Barbara O'Neill provides scientifically grounded explanations for the use of particular herbs, bridging the gap between traditional herbal wisdom and modern scientific understanding. Here are some of her insights:

Echinacea for Immune Support: Barbara explains that echinacea, a well-known immune-boosting herb, contains bioactive compounds like alkamides and polysaccharides. These compounds stimulate the immune system by increasing the production of white blood cells, thereby enhancing the body's ability to defend against infections. Scientific studies have corroborated echinacea's immunomodulatory effects.

Turmeric for Inflammation: Turmeric, with its active compound curcumin, is often recommended by Barbara for its anti-inflammatory properties. She highlights that curcumin inhibits inflammatory pathways at a molecular level by blocking molecules that trigger inflammation. Numerous scientific studies have substantiated turmeric's efficacy in managing chronic inflammation.

Ginger for Digestion: Barbara's insights into ginger's digestive benefits are supported by science. Gingerols, the bioactive compounds in ginger, stimulate the production of digestive enzymes, promoting smoother digestion. Studies have also shown ginger's effectiveness in reducing nausea and alleviating gastrointestinal discomfort.

Valerian for Sleep: When discussing valerian for sleep support, Barbara points to valerenic acid as the key compound. Valerian interacts with neurotransmitters in the brain, such as GABA, to induce a calming effect and improve sleep quality. Scientific research has demonstrated valerian's potential as a natural sleep aid.

Milk Thistle for Liver Health: Barbara emphasizes milk thistle's hepatoprotective properties. Silymarin, the active component in milk thistle, has antioxidant and anti-inflammatory effects that help protect liver cells from damage. Clinical studies have confirmed milk thistle's efficacy in supporting liver health.

St. John's Wort for Mood: Barbara discusses St. John's Wort as a natural remedy for mood disorders. Hypericin and hyperforin are the compounds responsible for its antidepressant effects. They work by modulating neurotransmitters like serotonin. Extensive research has validated St. John's Wort as a potential treatment for mild to moderate depression.

Lavender for Stress: Lavender, often recommended by Barbara for stress relief, contains linalool and linalyl acetate, compounds with soothing properties. They interact with receptors in the brain to reduce stress and anxiety. Clinical trials have shown lavender's efficacy in promoting relaxation.

Garlic for Cardiovascular Health: Barbara's insights into garlic's cardiovascular benefits are corroborated by scientific evidence. Allicin, a compound in garlic, has vasodilatory effects that help lower blood pressure. Garlic also improves cholesterol profiles and reduces the risk of heart disease.

Barbara O'Neill's ability to bridge traditional herbal knowledge with scientific explanations underscores the credibility and efficacy of herbal remedies. Her teachings empower individuals to make informed choices about their health by understanding the science behind the herbs they use.

Infusions and Decoctions

Infusions and decoctions are two essential techniques in herbalism for extracting the medicinal properties of plants. They are distinct methods of preparation, each suited for different types of plant materials and therapeutic purposes.

Infusions, often referred to as herbal teas, are a gentle way of extracting the delicate compounds found in herbs. This method is typically used for the aerial parts of plants, such as leaves and flowers. To create an infusion, one pours freshly boiled water over the chosen herbs, allowing them to steep for a specific duration, usually between 5 to 15 minutes. Infusions are known for their pleasant taste and are commonly consumed for both their flavor and therapeutic benefits. They work well with herbs containing essential oils, flavonoids, and volatile constituents.

On the other hand, decoctions are a more robust method of herbal preparation, primarily employed for tougher plant parts like roots, bark, seeds, and woody stems. Creating a decoction involves boiling the plant material in water. Unlike infusions, decoctions require an extended cooking time, ranging from 15 minutes to an hour, as the goal is to extract the medicinal compounds from these hardier plant parts. Decoctions are less about taste and more about harnessing the therapeutic properties of the herbs. They are often used for herbs that address chronic conditions or those with immune-boosting effects.

In summary, infusions and decoctions are distinct methods in herbalism, with infusions being ideal for delicate plant parts and pleasant-tasting herbal teas, while decoctions are suited for tougher plant materials and require boiling to extract their therapeutic compounds. The choice between these two methods depends on the type of herbs used and the desired therapeutic effects.

Infusion	Preparation	Effect	Barbara's Insights
Peppermint Infusion	Steep peppermint leaves in boiling water for 5-10 minutes.	Peppermint infusion aids digestion, relieves headaches, and promotes relaxation.	Barbara recommends peppermint infusion for digestive issues and relaxation.
Chamomile Infusion	Steep chamomile flowers in boiling water for 5-10 minutes.	Chamomile infusion has calming effects, relieves stress, and aids sleep.	Barbara suggests chamomile infusion for stress relief and better sleep.
Lemon Balm Infusion	Steep lemon balm leaves in boiling water for 5-10 minutes.	Lemon balm infusion supports mood, reduces anxiety, and improves cognitive function.	Barbara emphasizes the mood-enhancing effects of lemon balm infusion.
Ginger Infusion	Boil ginger root slices in water for 10-15 minutes.	Ginger infusion is anti-inflammatory, helps with nausea, and boosts the immune system.	Barbara highlights ginger infusion's anti-inflammatory properties and immune support.

Nettle Infusion	Steep nettle leaves in boiling water for 5-10 minutes.	Nettle infusion is rich in nutrients, supports detoxification, and provides energy.	Barbara mentions nettle infusion as a nutrient-rich option for detox and energy.

Here are some more specific tips and tricks for preparing herbal infusions:

Choose Wisely: Select herbs that align with your desired health benefits or flavor preferences.

Water Temperature Matters: Different herbs require different water temperatures. Use boiling water for robust herbs and slightly cooler water for delicate ones.

Cover While Steeping: Always cover your infusion as it steeps to trap the essential oils and prevent heat loss.

Timing is Key: Steeping times vary, so be precise. Over-steeping can lead to bitterness, while under-steeping may result in a weak infusion.

Experiment with Ratios: Adjust the herb-to-water ratio to control the strength of your infusion.

Mind the Pot: If using a teapot, make sure it's pre-warmed to maintain the infusion's temperature.

Strain Thoughtfully: Choose the right strainer or infuser to avoid bits of herbs in your cup.

Enhance the Flavor: Add natural sweeteners or complementary herbs and spices to suit your taste.

Temperature Transition: Rapidly cool down hot infusions for iced drinks by pouring over ice or refrigerating.

Storage Wisdom: Refrigerate leftover infusions promptly and consume within a day.

Blend and Enjoy: Create unique blends of herbs for delightful flavor combinations.

Consider Health Benefits: Be aware of the potential health advantages associated with the herbs you use.

Savor the Moment: Take time to appreciate the aroma and taste of your infusion for a relaxing experience.

Decoction	Preparation	Effects	Barbara's Insights
Dandelion Root Decoction	Boil dandelion root in water for 15-20 minutes, then strain.	Detoxifies the liver, supports digestion, and aids in kidney health.	Dandelion root decoction is excellent for detoxifying the liver and promoting overall digestive health.
Nettle Leaf Decoction	Steep nettle leaves in hot water for 10-15 minutes.	Rich in nutrients, supports the immune system, and promotes overall health.	Nettle leaf decoction is a nutritional powerhouse that supports the immune system and general well-being.
Echinacea Root Decoction	Simmer echinacea root in water for 20-30 minutes, then strain.	Boosts the immune system and helps fight infections and colds.	Echinacea root decoction is a potent immune booster, especially during cold and flu seasons.
Ginger Root Decoction	Boil ginger root in water for 15-20 minutes, then strain.	Aids digestion, reduces inflammation, and supports immune health.	Ginger root decoction aids digestion and can be soothing for the stomach.
Chamomile Flower Decoction	Steep chamomile flowers in hot water for 10-15 minutes.	Calms nerves, promotes relaxation, and aids in better sleep.	Chamomile flower decoction is a calming herbal remedy, ideal for relaxation and better sleep.

Here are some specific tips and tricks for preparing herbal decoctions:

Herb Selection: Choose the herbs that are best suited for decoctions, typically tougher parts like roots, bark, and seeds.

Cutting and Crushing: To increase the surface area for extraction, cut or crush the herbs into smaller pieces.

Proper Measurement: Use the correct herb-to-water ratio for your specific herb to achieve the desired strength.

Cold Start: Begin with cold water and add the herbs. Slowly bring it to a boil and then reduce to a simmer.

Low Heat: Simmer the mixture on low heat for an extended period. Decoctions usually require longer cooking times compared to infusions.

Lid On: Cover the pot with a lid to minimize evaporation and retain the medicinal properties.

Stir Occasionally: Stirring prevents herbs from sticking to the bottom of the pot and ensures even extraction.

Timing Matters: Decoctions can take anywhere from 20 minutes to an hour or more. Follow the recommended time for the herb you're using.

Straining Carefully: Once done, strain the liquid from the herb material, pressing to extract as much liquid as possible.

Cool Gradually: Allow the decoction to cool gradually before transferring it to a container.

Storage and Consumption: Store any leftover decoction in the refrigerator and use within a day or as recommended.

Flavor Enhancement: You can improve the taste by adding natural sweeteners or complementary herbs and spices.

Herbal Knowledge: Be aware of the specific health benefits associated with the herbs you're using in your decoction.

Tinctures and Extracts

Tinctures and extracts are concentrated liquid forms of herbal remedies, each with its own method of preparation and specific uses.

A tincture is typically made by soaking a specific herb or combination of herbs in alcohol or another solvent. This allows the alcohol to extract the active compounds and beneficial properties of the herbs, resulting in a potent and concentrated liquid. Tinctures are known for their long shelf life, often lasting for several years, and they are usually administered in drop form. The alcohol acts as a preservative and helps to maintain the potency of the herbal remedy.

On the other hand, extracts are created by using a solvent, such as water or glycerin, to draw out the beneficial components of herbs. Unlike tinctures, extracts do not contain alcohol. Glycerin extracts, in particular, are a suitable alternative for individuals who wish to avoid alcohol in their herbal remedies. These extracts are often used for children or individuals with alcohol sensitivities.

Both tinctures and extracts are highly concentrated forms of herbal medicines, which means that a small amount can be quite powerful. They are typically used for therapeutic purposes, such as addressing specific health issues or promoting overall well-being. When preparing tinctures and extracts, it's crucial to use high-quality herbs and follow precise guidelines to ensure the effectiveness and safety of the final product.

Barbara O'Neill often emphasizes the importance of using tinctures and extracts as part of a holistic approach to health and healing. She suggests that these concentrated herbal forms can be valuable tools in addressing various health conditions and promoting overall vitality when used in conjunction with a balanced diet and other natural remedies. Her insights often revolve around the idea that these concentrated forms of herbs can provide targeted support for specific health concerns, making them a valuable addition to a holistic wellness regimen.

Tincture	Preparation	Effect	Barbara Insights
Valerian Tincture	Tincture: 1:2 in 40% alcohol, 40-90 drops before bed	Sedative, relaxes the nervous system, promotes sleep	Valerian tincture is a natural remedy for sleep disorders and anxiety. It helps calm the nerves and promote restful sleep.
Milk Thistle Tincture	Tincture: 1:2 in 50% alcohol, 20-60 drops daily	Supports liver health, detoxifies the liver, aids digestion	Milk thistle tincture is beneficial for liver health and detoxification. It supports the liver in processing toxins and aids in digestion.
Echinacea Tincture	Tincture: 1:2 in 40% alcohol, 20-40 drops 2-3 times daily	Boosts the immune system, fights infections, reduces inflammation	Echinacea tincture is known for its immune-boosting properties. It helps the body fight off infections and reduces inflammation.
Chamomile Tincture	Tincture: 1:2 in 30% alcohol, 20-40 drops as needed	Calms nerves, relieves anxiety, aids digestion	Chamomile tincture is a gentle remedy for calming nerves and reducing anxiety. It also aids in digestion and soothes the stomach.
Ginger Tincture	Tincture: 1:2 in 40% alcohol, 30-60 drops as needed	Supports digestion, relieves nausea, reduces inflammation	Ginger tincture is excellent for supporting digestion, relieving nausea, and reducing inflammation in the body.

Here's a list of essential items you'll need to start making tinctures and extracts:

Herbs: Choose the herbs you want to work with based on your specific needs and preferences.

Dried Herbs: Many tinctures and extracts are made from dried herbs. Ensure you have a good supply.

Fresh Herbs (Optional): Some tinctures can be made from fresh herbs. If you prefer this method, you'll need access to fresh herbs.

Glass Jars with Lids: Use clean glass jars with tight-fitting lids for macerating herbs.

Alcohol (or Vinegar): High-proof alcohol, such as vodka or brandy, is commonly used for tinctures. Alternatively, you can use apple cider vinegar if you prefer a non-alcoholic option.

Distilled Water (Optional): For diluting tinctures if needed.

Cheesecloth or Fine Strainer: For straining the liquid from the herbs.

Dark Glass Bottles: To store the finished tinctures and extracts, use amber or dark glass bottles to protect them from light.

Labels: Clearly label your jars and bottles with the herb name, date of preparation, and any additional notes.

Funnel: Makes it easier to pour the tincture or extract into bottles without spilling.

Knife and Cutting Board: If you're using fresh herbs, you'll need these for chopping or crushing.

Measuring Tools: Use measuring cups or scales to ensure accurate measurements.

Pen and Notebook: Keep a notebook for recording your recipes, observations, and any adjustments you make.

Storage Area: Find a cool, dark place to store your tinctures and extracts while they macerate.

Patience: Tinctures and extracts require time to macerate and develop their full potency. Be patient and allow them to sit for several weeks.

Remember to work in a clean and organized environment to maintain the quality and effectiveness of your tinctures and extracts. Additionally, familiarize yourself with the specific herbs you're using, as their properties and recommended preparation methods may vary.

Herbal Treatments for Common Ailments

Barbara O'Neill, an esteemed herbalist and holistic health expert, has dedicated her life to unraveling the secrets of these botanical marvels and sharing her wisdom with the world.

Imagine a world where minor ailments like headaches, indigestion, or sleep disturbances can be effectively managed with the gentle touch of nature. It's a world that Barbara O'Neill invites us to explore, where herbs serve as allies in our quest for well-being.

One common ailment that often plagues us is the dreaded headache. Instead of reaching for over-the-counter pain relievers, Barbara suggests turning to feverfew, a herbaceous plant known for its ability to alleviate migraines and tension headaches. Its active compound, parthenolide, helps reduce inflammation in blood vessels, which can be a primary trigger for headaches. By incorporating feverfew into our lives, we may find respite from those throbbing pains that disrupt our day.

Indigestion, another widespread concern, finds its nemesis in the soothing embrace of peppermint. Barbara O'Neill extols the virtues of this aromatic herb, which contains menthol, a compound that relaxes the muscles of the gastrointestinal tract. A warm cup of peppermint tea post-meal can work wonders in calming an upset stomach, making dining a more enjoyable experience.

And when the hustle and bustle of daily life leaves us tossing and turning at night, Barbara offers a remedy rooted in centuries of tradition – valerian. This herb, known for its sedative properties, aids in improving sleep quality and reducing the time it takes to fall asleep. Just a few drops of valerian tincture before bedtime can usher in a night of restful slumber.

But it's not only physical ailments that Barbara addresses; she recognizes the profound connection between our emotional well-being and our physical health. Anxiety, a prevalent modern affliction, can be tempered with the grace of lavender. Barbara encourages the use of lavender essential oil, which, when inhaled or applied topically, has been shown to reduce anxiety levels and promote relaxation. In the world of herbs, sometimes it's the gentlest scents that wield the mightiest powers.

This journey through herbal treatments for common ailments serves as a testament to Barbara O'Neill's unwavering commitment to holistic health. It's a journey that reminds us of the immense wisdom contained in nature's pharmacy, waiting to be harnessed for our healing. As we embrace these natural remedies, we not only alleviate our ailments but also reconnect with the timeless traditions of herbal medicine, guided by the sage wisdom of Barbara O'Neill.

In our pursuit of well-being through herbal treatments for common ailments, we uncover a rich tapestry of natural solutions that span the spectrum of human health. Barbara O'Neill, an holistic health and herbal medicine luminary, beckons us to delve deeper into this world of botanical wonders.

Picture a scenario where seasonal allergies, with their sneezes and sniffles, no longer hold us hostage. Barbara introduces us to the humble but potent nettle leaf, a herbal ally renowned for its ability to combat allergies. Nettle leaf contains histamine, which may seem counterintuitive given that histamine is often associated with allergic reactions. However, when consumed in the form of nettle tea or tincture, it can actually help to alleviate allergy symptoms by blocking the body's histamine receptors. It's a testament to nature's ability to provide solutions even for conditions it seemingly contributes to.

Digestive discomfort is a universal concern, but instead of relying on antacids, Barbara advocates for the use of slippery elm bark. This herbal remedy forms a soothing gel when mixed with water, which can help alleviate the irritation of the digestive tract. Whether it's heartburn, gastritis, or even irritable bowel syndrome, slippery elm bark offers a gentle touch to ease discomfort.

Many women turn to red raspberry leaf tea during pregnancy, believing it can help tone the uterine muscles and potentially ease labor. While scientific research on this is limited, the wisdom of generations of midwives and herbalists speaks to its value.

The stresses of modern life can sometimes lead to adrenal fatigue, a condition where the body's stress response system becomes compromised. Barbara recommends the adaptogenic herb ashwagandha as a potential solution. This remarkable herb is believed to support the adrenal glands, helping the body better cope with stress. In a world where stress is often a constant companion, ashwagandha offers respite.

And then there's the often overlooked but vital aspect of oral health. Barbara shares insights into the use of myrrh resin, which has been employed for centuries to maintain healthy gums and teeth. Myrrh possesses antimicrobial properties that can help combat oral bacteria and promote oral hygiene. It's a reminder that the world of herbal medicine extends even to the care of our pearly whites.

As we journey deeper into the field of herbal treatments, we are not merely addressing physical ailments; we are nurturing a profound connection with the natural world. Barbara O'Neill's wisdom serves as a guiding light, illuminating the path to holistic health through the gifts of nature. Each herb we explore becomes a thread in the tapestry of our well-being, a testament to the incredible synergy between humanity and the botanical territory.

Herbal Treatment	Common Ailment	Barbara's Insights
Nettle Leaf	Seasonal Allergies	Nettle leaf contains histamine, which, when consumed, can alleviate allergy symptoms by blocking histamine receptors.
Slippery Elm Bark	Digestive Discomfort	Slippery elm bark forms a soothing gel when mixed with water, helping to ease digestive tract irritation, including heartburn and gastritis.
Red Raspberry Leaf	Women's Health	Red raspberry leaf is considered a uterine tonic and is often used during pregnancy to potentially tone uterine muscles and ease labor.
Ashwagandha	Adrenal Fatigue	Ashwagandha is an adaptogenic herb believed to support the adrenal glands, helping the body cope with stress and adrenal fatigue.
Myrrh Resin	Oral Health	Myrrh resin possesses antimicrobial properties that can combat oral bacteria, promoting healthy gums and teeth.

Bonus #2: Video Tutorial for Herbal Remedies

As you delve into the captivating pages of "Dr. Barbara Bible," I'm delighted to offer you an exclusive bonus that broadens your learning experience far beyond the traditional confines of text. Hidden within this note is a special QR code, a gateway to a rich array of practical knowledge in the realm of natural healing.

This QR code leads you to a carefully curated collection of video recipes, designed to guide you through the creation of Herbal Infusions, Decoctions, Tinctures, and Extracts. These aren't just instructional videos; they represent a voyage into the core of herbal medicine, illuminating age-old practices that have fostered health and well-being across generations. Scanning this QR code transports you into a realm where the venerable art of herbal remedies becomes a tangible part of your life. Regardless of your experience level in herbal crafting, from beginners to experts, these videos provide insightful, step-by-step guidance that easily integrates into your wellness practices.

This bonus goes beyond being a mere supplement to the book. It represents our dedication to offering a comprehensive and engaging educational experience. It's a chance for you to witness how nature's offerings are transformed into powerful healing agents, to understand the nuances of selecting and preparing herbs, and to learn about maintaining their therapeutic qualities.

We encourage you to embark on this exploration with an eager heart and an inquisitive mind, delving into the hands-on aspects of herbal medicine. Let these video recipes accompany you on your path to mastering the art of natural healing, broadening your horizons, and enriching your practice.

Thus, please proceed to scan the QR code and enter a world where the time-honored tradition of herbal healing is at your fingertips. May these videos serve as a source of inspiration and knowledge, contributing significantly to your health and wellness.

@YOURHEALINGHERBS

Chapter 5: Diabetes Management

How to Impact on Diabetes

In this extensive section, we explore the impact of diet on diabetes management, drawing upon the teachings of Dr. Barbara O'Neill. Her insights provide a comprehensive understanding of how dietary choices can influence the body's energy production, blood glucose levels, and overall health, especially in the context of diabetes management.

Dr. O'Neill highlights the critical role of oxygen in the body's energy production. The metabolic pathway that utilizes oxygen produces significantly more energy, yielding about 36 units of energy, in stark contrast to the pathway that operates without oxygen, which generates only 2 units. This disparity underscores the importance of a diet that supports the body's oxygen-utilizing metabolic processes. Foods rich in nutrients that enhance oxygenation and energy production are crucial for maintaining high energy levels and efficient bodily functions, particularly for individuals managing diabetes.

The type of carbohydrates consumed plays a vital role in managing blood glucose levels. Dr. O'Neill draws attention to the differences between amylopectin A and amylopectin C. Amylopectin C, found in foods like chickpeas, lentils, and other beans, leads to a more gradual and consistent rise in blood glucose levels. This is in contrast to amylopectin A, which can cause rapid spikes in blood sugar. For diabetes management, maintaining steady blood glucose levels is essential, and incorporating foods with amylopectin C can be beneficial in achieving this balance.

A key component of Dr. O'Neill's dietary recommendations for diabetes management is the emphasis on high-fiber plant-based foods. These foods, along with protein sources like beans and nuts, and healthy fats such as coconut oil, contribute to a balanced diet. High-fiber foods help in regulating blood sugar levels, while proteins and healthy fats provide sustained energy and satiety, helping to prevent overeating and manage weight – both crucial aspects of diabetes management.

Coconut oil is lauded by Dr. O'Neill as one of the best oils for cooking. Its stability, attributed to the absence of double bonds, prevents deterioration under heat. This stability makes it a healthier choice compared to oils that can form harmful compounds when heated. Using coconut oil in cooking can be part of a healthy dietary regimen, supporting overall wellness and effective diabetes management.

Dr. O'Neill often references the ancient wisdom of Hippocrates: "Let food be your medicine and medicine be your food." This statement encapsulates the core belief that the body has a remarkable capacity for self-healing, and that diet plays a crucial role in this process. Embracing a diet that is rich in whole, nutrient-dense foods can significantly aid in the body's natural healing processes, especially important for those managing chronic conditions like diabetes.

In summary, Dr. Barbara O'Neill's teachings offer a holistic perspective on managing diabetes through dietary choices. Understanding the nuances of how different foods affect energy production, blood glucose levels, and overall health is key to effective diabetes management. Her approach encourages a return to natural, whole foods, and recognizes the power of nutrition in supporting the body's inherent healing abilities. By adopting these principles, individuals with diabetes can better manage their condition, enhancing their overall health and quality of life.

Exercise and Diabetes

Dr. O'Neill posits that high-intensity interval training can be markedly more effective in managing diabetes than traditional, moderate exercises like a 1-hour walk. HIIT, characterized by short bursts of intense activity followed by periods of rest, has been shown to significantly improve insulin sensitivity and glucose metabolism. This type of training challenges the body in a way that can lead to more substantial metabolic changes, making it a potent tool in the diabetic management toolkit.

The benefits of HIIT extend beyond just glucose metabolism. Dr. O'Neill points out that movie stars often pay hefty sums for human growth hormone (HGH) therapies, known for their anti-aging and metabolism-boosting effects. However, HIIT can stimulate the natural production of HGH in the body. Engaging in just 50 minutes of HIIT daily can yield benefits comparable to those of expensive HGH treatments, making it an accessible and cost-effective method to improve health and manage diabetes.

One of the most striking benefits of HIIT, as noted by Dr. O'Neill, is its ability to reverse insulin resistance in a remarkably short time. Studies have shown that engaging in HIIT can lead to significant improvements in insulin sensitivity within just one week. This rapid response highlights the incredible efficacy of exercise in combating one of the primary underlying issues in diabetes - insulin resistance.

Dr. O'Neill emphasizes the combination of reduced insulin intake and high-intensity exercise as a strategy for managing blood glucose levels in individuals with diabetes. This approach not only helps in controlling blood sugar but also reduces the dependency on external insulin, thereby promoting a more natural regulation of glucose levels in the body.

An illustrative example provided by Dr. O'Neill involves the use of rebounding exercise, a form of exercise involving a mini-trampoline, combined with specific dietary modifications. She cites a case where an individual was able to reduce their insulin intake dramatically - from 40 units to just 10 units daily - within two weeks. This case study exemplifies the synergistic effect of combining exercise with dietary changes, showcasing how lifestyle modifications can lead to significant improvements in diabetes management.

In conclusion, Dr. Barbara O'Neill's approach to managing diabetes through exercise, particularly high-intensity interval training, offers a dynamic and effective alternative to traditional methods. Her emphasis on the power of exercise to enhance insulin sensitivity and promote natural hormone production presents a compelling argument for incorporating HIIT into diabetes management strategies. Coupled with dietary changes, this approach can lead to substantial improvements in blood glucose control and overall health, offering a beacon of hope for individuals navigating the challenges of diabetes.

Q&A

How do I find more resources on diabetes management and view Barbara O'Neill's past lectures?

— For a deeper understanding of diabetes and to access Barbara O'Neill's previous presentations, various resources are available. You can reach out via the church's email for specific inquiries or educational materials. Additionally, her past lectures and seminars can be found on live stream channels and YouTube, offering a wealth of information on diabetes management and other health-related topics.

What are the dietary recommendations for controlling blood sugar levels?

— To effectively regulate blood sugar levels, certain foods should be limited or avoided. These include high-glycemic items like breakfast cereals, bread, cakes, biscuits, pies, pizza, pasta, rice, potatoes, and sugar. These foods are quickly broken down into glucose in the gastrointestinal tract, leading to spikes in blood sugar levels. Opting for low-glycemic alternatives and incorporating more whole, unprocessed foods into your diet can be beneficial in maintaining stable glucose levels.

Can you explain the function of insulin in blood sugar regulation?

— Insulin is a vital hormone in the regulation of blood glucose levels. Its primary function is to facilitate the transportation of glucose from the bloodstream into the body's cells, where it is used for energy. When the body becomes resistant to insulin, a condition known as insulin resistance, it can lead to elevated blood sugar levels and eventually result in diabetes mellitus. Understanding and managing insulin sensitivity is therefore crucial in the prevention and treatment of diabetes.

In what ways does high-intensity interval training (HIIT) impact diabetes?

— High-intensity interval training, a form of exercise characterized by short bursts of intense activity followed by rest periods, can have a significant positive impact on diabetes management. HIIT works by depleting glycogen stores in the cells, which can lead to a reversal of insulin resistance. This type of training not only improves overall fitness but also aids in better glucose regulation, making it a valuable component in the management of diabetes.

What diet modifications are beneficial for managing diabetes?

— Managing diabetes effectively often involves making specific dietary changes. Consuming a diet high in fiber, rich in protein, and including healthy fats, when combined with high-intensity interval training, can lead to weight loss and improved metabolic health. Such a diet can also stimulate the release of the human growth hormone, which not only slows down the aging process but also enhances circulation to the skin. These dietary modifications, along with regular physical activity, can significantly aid in the control of diabetes and improve overall health.

Chapter 6: Water Therapy

Barbara O'Neill, in her teachings on natural health and wellness, discusses a unique approach known as "water therapy." This therapy, also sometimes referred to as hydrotherapy, is based on the use of water in various forms and temperatures to promote health and healing. Here's an overview of the key concepts and practices associated with water therapy as advocated by Barbara O'Neill.

Contrast Showers or Baths

Contrast showers or baths, a key component of water therapy as advocated by Barbara O'Neill, are an intriguing and accessible method for enhancing health and vitality. This practice involves alternating between hot and cold water during showers or baths, leveraging the unique properties of temperature to benefit the body.

The underlying principle of contrast showers or baths is rooted in the body's response to different temperatures. When exposed to hot water, the blood vessels in the skin and superficial tissues dilate or widen. This dilation increases blood flow to the skin and muscles, bringing warmth and nutrients while also facilitating the removal of metabolic waste. The warmth of the water can also help relax muscles and soothe aches, leading to a reduction in muscle tension and promoting a sense of relaxation.

In contrast, exposure to cold water causes vasoconstriction, the narrowing of blood vessels. This reaction reduces blood flow to the skin's surface, redirecting it to the core of the body. The immediate effect is a feeling of invigoration, as the body experiences a rush of adrenaline. This switch to cold water also stimulates the nervous system, leading to increased alertness and clarity of mind.

Health Benefits of Contrast Showers or Baths

Enhanced Circulation: The alternation between hot and cold water creates a kind of 'vascular gymnastics' in the body. The hot water causes vasodilation, followed by vasoconstriction due to the cold. This rhythmic change in blood vessel diameter enhances blood circulation throughout the body, which is beneficial for cardiovascular health and can aid in faster recovery from muscle soreness.

Detoxification: Improved circulation also plays a key role in detoxification. Enhanced blood flow ensures that waste products from cellular metabolism are efficiently transported to excretory organs. The lymphatic system, crucial for removing toxins, also benefits from the improved circulation, thus supporting the body's natural detoxification processes.

Immune System Boost: Regularly engaging in contrast showers can bolster the immune system. The cold phase of the shower stimulates leukocytes, which are immune cells that fight infection. This increased activity can lead to a stronger immune system, potentially reducing the frequency and severity of illnesses.

Mental Health and Vitality: The stimulating effect of cold water, coupled with the relaxing properties of hot water, can have a positive impact on mental health. The practice has been associated with reduced stress levels, improved mood, and increased mental alertness. The endorphin rush triggered by the cold water can also provide a natural boost to one's mood and energy levels.

Skin and Hair Health: Contrast showers can also benefit skin and hair health. The cold water phase helps to tighten and constrict blood flow, reducing inflammation and puffiness in the skin. It can also close the pores and cuticles of the hair, leading to smoother, shinier hair. On the other hand, the hot water phase opens pores, helping to cleanse the skin and remove impurities.

Practical Tips for Contrast Showers or Baths

Starting Slowly: For beginners, it's important to start slowly and gradually adjust to the temperature changes. Begin with a comfortable warm temperature and slowly introduce cooler temperatures.

Duration and Frequency: The duration of each hot and cold phase can vary based on individual tolerance, but a general guideline is to aim for about 1-2 minutes of hot water followed by 30 seconds to 1 minute of cold water. Repeat this cycle for the duration of the shower. Consistency is key; practicing contrast showers regularly can enhance the benefits.

Safety Considerations: It's important to listen to your body and avoid extremes in temperature, especially if you have health conditions such as cardiovascular issues. Pregnant women and individuals with certain medical conditions should consult a healthcare professional before starting contrast showers.

Ending on Cold: Many practitioners recommend ending the shower on a cold cycle. This leaves the body invigorated and stimulates the immune system, providing a refreshing and energizing start to the day.

Contrast showers or baths can be a simple yet effective addition to a holistic health routine. When combined with other healthful practices such as a balanced diet, regular exercise, and stress management techniques, they can significantly contribute to overall well-being.

In summary, contrast showers or baths present a unique and practical method to enhance physical and mental health. This simple practice, accessible to most, harnesses the power of water and temperature to invigorate the body, boost health, and elevate vitality. By regularly incorporating this into one's routine, individuals can experience a range of benefits from improved circulation and detoxification to enhanced immune function and increased mental clarity.

Steam Inhalation

Steam inhalation, a therapeutic practice championed by Barbara O'Neill, is an ancient and natural remedy, especially beneficial for respiratory health. The process involves inhaling warm, moist air, which can be infused with natural herbs or essential oils for added benefits. This simple yet effective treatment offers a range of health benefits, particularly for the respiratory system.

The practice of steam inhalation typically involves boiling water and allowing the steam to rise while the individual leans over the container, inhaling the warm vapors. Often, a towel is draped over the head and the container to create a small enclosure, enhancing the effectiveness of the inhalation process. The temperature should be warm enough to create steam but not so hot as to burn the skin or the respiratory tract.

Benefits of Steam Inhalation

Opens Nasal Passages: The warm, moist air from steam inhalation works effectively to open nasal passages. This is particularly beneficial for individuals suffering from conditions like sinusitis or a common cold, where nasal congestion is a primary symptom.
Facilitates Easier Breathing: For those with respiratory issues such as bronchitis, asthma, or a common cold, steam inhalation can facilitate easier breathing. The warm steam helps to moisten the airways, easing the process of breathing in individuals with respiratory distress.
Loosens Mucus and Phlegm: Steam inhalation is effective in loosening mucus and phlegm in the lungs and nasal passages. This loosening helps in clearing the airways, thus providing relief from congestion and making it easier to expel mucus through coughing or blowing the nose.
Soothing Effect on Irritated Throat: The warm steam provides a soothing effect on an irritated or sore throat, which is often a symptom of a cold or other respiratory infection. It helps in hydrating and calming the throat lining.
Enhances Sinus Health: Regular steam inhalation can improve overall sinus health, helping to prevent the recurrence of sinus issues. It keeps the mucosal lining in the sinuses moist, which is essential for the proper functioning of the sinuses.

Adding Herbs and Essential Oils

Enhancing the steam inhalation process with herbs and essential oils can provide additional therapeutic benefits:

- **Eucalyptus Oil**: Known for its decongestant properties, eucalyptus oil can be added to the water for steam inhalation. It helps in clearing the nasal passages and has antimicrobial properties.
- **Peppermint Oil**: This oil has menthol, which can help in opening the breathing passages and relieving congestion.
- **Lavender Oil**: Renowned for its calming properties, lavender oil can be added to provide a relaxing and soothing experience, especially beneficial before bedtime.
- **Chamomile**: Known for its anti-inflammatory properties, chamomile can be soothing for irritated mucous membranes.

Safety Considerations

While steam inhalation is generally safe, certain precautions should be taken:
- Ensure that the water is not too hot to prevent burns.
- Individuals with certain health conditions, such as heart problems, central nervous system disorders, or pregnant women, should consult with a healthcare provider before starting steam inhalation therapy.
- Essential oils should be used cautiously, as some individuals may have allergic reactions to specific oils.

Steam inhalation can be a valuable addition to a holistic approach to health. When combined with a healthy lifestyle, adequate hydration, and a balanced diet, it can significantly contribute to respiratory health and overall well-being. It's a simple, natural remedy that aligns with Barbara O'Neill's philosophy of using nature's tools to support the body's healing processes. In summary, steam inhalation is a time-tested, natural method for alleviating respiratory discomfort and enhancing sinus and lung health. By understanding and utilizing this simple technique, individuals can take an active role in managing their respiratory health, in line with Barbara O'Neill's teachings on the power of natural therapies.

Foot Baths

Foot baths, an integral part of water therapy as highlighted by Barbara O'Neill, represent a simple yet profoundly therapeutic practice. The concept of soaking feet in hot water, enhanced with herbs or salts, offers more than just immediate relaxation; it taps into the deeper healing properties of water and natural additives.

A foot bath involves immersing the feet in a basin of hot water. The temperature should be comfortably warm but not scalding, typically around 100-110°F (37-43°C). This practice can be an incredibly soothing experience, particularly after extended periods of standing, walking, or physical exertion.

Health Benefits of Foot Baths

Improved Circulation: The warmth from the hot water helps to expand blood vessels in the feet, enhancing blood flow. This improved circulation can help to alleviate conditions like cold feet or numbness and can also aid in faster recovery from foot injuries.

Stress Reduction: Foot baths are known for their ability to induce deep relaxation and reduce stress. The warmth and comfort provided by the water can help to soothe the entire nervous system, promoting a sense of calm and relaxation.

Pain Relief: For those suffering from foot pain, whether due to conditions like arthritis or simply from day-to-day activities, a warm foot bath can provide significant pain relief. The heat helps to relax the muscles and alleviate tension in the feet.

Detoxification: Adding certain salts or herbs to a foot bath can enhance its detoxifying properties. Ingredients like Epsom salt are known to help draw out toxins from the body through the feet, aiding in overall detoxification.

Enhanced Sleep Quality: Engaging in a foot bath before bedtime can improve sleep quality. The relaxation effect of the warm water helps to prepare the body for sleep, making it easier to fall asleep and enjoy a more restful night.

Adding Herbs and Salts for Additional Benefits

Epsom Salt: Rich in magnesium, Epsom salt can help reduce inflammation, relieve muscle cramps, and improve nerve function. It's also beneficial for skin health, helping to soften and exfoliate the skin on the feet.

Lavender: Known for its calming properties, adding lavender to a foot bath can enhance relaxation and stress relief. It's particularly useful for those with sleep difficulties.

Peppermint: For a refreshing and invigorating foot bath, peppermint is an excellent choice. It can help rejuvenate tired feet and has natural cooling properties.

Chamomile: Chamomile, with its anti-inflammatory and soothing properties, can be particularly beneficial for those with skin irritations or dry skin on their feet.

Tea Tree Oil: Recognized for its antifungal and antibacterial properties, tea tree oil is a great addition for foot health, particularly for those prone to fungal infections like athlete's foot.

Practical Tips for Foot Baths

Duration: A typical foot bath should last between 15-30 minutes to allow enough time for the body to reap the benefits.

Water Level: The water should be deep enough to cover the feet completely. This ensures that all parts of the feet, including the ankles, receive the therapeutic benefits.

Temperature Check: Always check the water temperature before immersing your feet to prevent burns.

Frequency: Regular foot baths can be a beneficial addition to a wellness routine. Even a couple of times a week can provide significant health benefits.

Post-Bath Care: After a foot bath, it's important to rinse the feet with clean water and dry them thoroughly, especially between the toes, to prevent any fungal growth.

Foot baths can easily be incorporated into a holistic health routine. They are a simple, accessible form of self-care that can have profound effects on overall well-being. When combined with other health practices like proper nutrition, adequate hydration, and regular physical activity, foot baths can contribute significantly to a balanced and healthy lifestyle.

In summary, the practice of foot baths, as advocated by Barbara O'Neill, is a testament to the power of simple, natural methods in promoting health and well-being. By embracing this practice, individuals can experience a range of benefits from improved circulation and stress relief to enhanced sleep quality and detoxification, all contributing to a more balanced and healthful life.

Conclusion

As we draw the curtains on the enriching book that "Dr. Barbara Bible" has been, it's important to pause and reflect on the profound insights and transformative knowledge that Simon Jr. Jackson has meticulously woven into the fabric of this book. This literary odyssey, a tribute to the pioneering spirit of Dr. Barbara O'Neill, serves not just as a repository of knowledge but as a beacon guiding us toward a more harmonious and healthful existence.

Throughout the chapters, we've delved deep into the essence of holistic health, uncovering the layers of nutrition, detoxification, herbal remedies, and the foundational pillars of a healthy lifestyle. Each page turned has offered not just information, but an invitation to embark on a personal path of health and self-discovery.

In a world often swayed by the allure of quick fixes and fleeting trends, "Dr. Barbara Bible" stands as a testament to the enduring wisdom of nature and the remarkable capabilities of our bodies to heal and thrive when given the right nurture and care. Barbara's philosophies, brought to life by Simon Jr. Jackson's eloquent prose, remind us that health is not a destination but something to travel through – one that is deeply personal, infinitely varied, and richly rewarding.

As you, dear reader, move forward from the final page of this book, it's hoped that the teachings of Dr. O'Neill, as presented by Simon Jr. Jackson, resonate within you, not just as words read but as wisdom lived. May the seeds of knowledge planted through these pages blossom into a life lived with vitality, purpose, and a profound connection to the healing powers of nature.

"Dr. Barbara Bible" is more than just a book; it's a companion for your route, a source of comfort during challenging times, and a reminder of the incredible power you hold over your health and well-being. As Barbara herself would advocate, let us not merely treat symptoms but nurture the whole self – mind, body, and spirit – embracing the beauty and balance of life, as nature intended.

In closing, let this book be a beginning, not an end – a starting point for a new life.

Made in United States
Troutdale, OR
03/05/2024

18236141R00058